THE PLEASURES AND PERILS OF GENIUS: MOSTLY MOZART

Mental Health Library Series

Monograph 2

edited by
George H. Pollock, M.D., Ph.D.

THE PLEASURES AND PERILS OF GENIUS: MOSTLY MOZART

Edited by
Peter Ostwald, M.D.
Leonard S. Zegans, M.D.

INTERNATIONAL UNIVERSITIES PRESS, INC.
Madison   Connecticut

Copyright © 1993, International Universities Press, Inc.

Library of Congress Cataloging-in-Publication Data

The Pleasures and perils of genius: mostly Mozart/edited by Peter
  Ostwald, Leonard S. Zegans.
    p. cm.—(Mental health library series; monograph 2)
    Includes bibliographical references and indexes.
    ISBN 0-8236-4162-7
    1. Mozart, Wolfgang Amadeus, 1756-1791—Psychology. 2. Genius.
I. Ostwald, Peter F. II. Zegans, Leonard S. III. Series.
ML410.M9P49 1993
780'.92—dc20   93-24461
                                                                   CIP
                                                                   MN

Manufactured in the United States of America

Contents

Contributors

Thomas Bauman, Ph.D.—Professor of Music, University of Washington, Seattle, Washington.

Clifford Cranna, Ph.D.—Musical Administrator, San Francisco Opera.

Peter J. Davies, M.D., F.R.A.C.P.—Private Practice Physician in Internal Medicine and Gastroenterology, Melbourne, Australia.

Stuart Feder, M.D.—Faculty, New York Psychoanalytic Institute.

David Henry Feldman, Ph.D.—Professor of Developmental Psychology, Eliot-Pearson Department of Child Study; and Director of the Developmental Science Group, Tufts University, Medford, Massachusetts.

Gary S. Gelber, M.D.—Associate Clinical Professor of Psychiatry and Psychiatrist, Health Program for Performing Artists, University of California, San Francisco.

Marc Gottlieb—Conductor, Tulsa Opera; Violinist; and Former Leader of the Claremont String Quartet.

Paul Hersh—Concert Pianist and Violist, San Francisco Conservatory of Music Faculty.

Hans Hotter—Eminent Bass-Baritone, now also a Master Teacher.

Lotfi Mansouri—General Director, San Francisco Opera.

Robert L. Marshall, Ph.D.—Louis, Frances, and Jeffrey Sachar Professor of Music, Brandeis University, Waltham, Massachusetts.

Lise Deschamps Ostwald—Pianist, Director of "Opera-Go-Round," San Francisco.

Peter Ostwald, M.D.—Professor of Psychiatry and Medical Director, Health Program for Performing Artists, University of California, San Francisco.

George H. Pollock, M.D., Ph.D.—Ruth and Evelyn Dunbar Distinguished Professor of Psychiatry and Behavioral Sciences, Northwestern University Medical School, Chicago, Illinois.

Günter B. Risse, M.D., Ph.D.—Professor and Chairman, Department of History of Health Sciences, University of California, San Francisco.

Erna Schwerin, M.A.—Clinical Psychologist; Founder and President, *Friends of Mozart*, New York.

Dean Keith Simonton, Ph.D.—Professor of Psychology, University of California, Davis.

Leonard S. Zegans, M.D.—Professor of Psychiatry and Director of Education, Langley Porter Psychiatric Institute, Department of Psychiatry, University of California, San Francisco.

Introduction

Few subjects have been more fascinating and more puzzling than that of genius, a very rare but very powerful human phenomenon. It seems that from time immemorial a person has suddenly come on the scene with incredibly superior mental abilities and the capacity to see things in a totally new way, to contribute useful and original things and ideas, and to change the course of history. Efforts to explain this phenomenon have ranged from the ancient approach of considering such people to be gods or godlike, through the idea that they are mentally abnormal, to the current view that they possess unique intelligence and a special character structure. Social conditions and historical trends are also felt to be significant in bringing to prominence the men and women who are ultimately called geniuses.

Being such a person highly endowed with unusual talents, strikingly different from ordinary or normal people, imposes great responsibilities as well as stresses, not only on the individuals themselves but also on those who are close to them, concerned about them, and interested in what they do, including members of their family, their friends, teachers, and colleagues. It has been observed that some of the people called geniuses seem to be quite self-centered, even narcissistic. Much of the time they may be totally absorbed in the work they are doing, so that little time, energy, or interest is invested in social relationships. Some men and women of genius seem out of step with their social environment. Others adhere to life styles that may seem troubled, even chaotic. From the viewpoint of practical clinical management, it has been observed that geniuses may be difficult patients who tend to direct their own treatment, to resist, or to try avoiding treatment altogether. An interesting current trend in conceptualizing the problem is to dismiss the very idea of genius as possibly too elitist, with the result that behavior of these highly exceptional people is reduced to more general categories such as "creativity" or "psychiatric disorder."

The present book is based on an interdisciplinary conference held at the University of California in San Francisco in 1991. The goal was to explore some of the advantages and disadvantages of being a genius. In doing so, and to bring things to a rather more concrete level, it was felt desirable that one particular genius, Wolfgang Amadeus Mozart, be the focus of attention.

It so happened that 1991 was a good year for Mozart, paradoxically since that year marked the two hundredth anniversary of his tragic and untimely death at age 35. There were Mozart festivals throughout the world that bicentennial year, and a great deal of his music was performed. New recordings and new books about him appeared. Yet the paradox of Mozart was not resolved. "We are drawn to him," wrote *New York Times* critic Edward Rothstein, "but he remains alien: he is in our world but not of it" (1991, p. 32). And in the background, of course, were the excitement and the questions raised by the very successful film *Amadeus*, portraying Mozart as an extraordinarily playful but maladroit, unsophisticated, even masochistic character victimized by Antonio Salieri.

Indeed, Mozart was one of the greatest child prodigies in recorded history. His incredible career had been guided and controlled by his musician-father until the younger man rebelled and ran into serious difficulty, partly because of his quirky personality, partly because of an unlucky marriage, and partly because of changing socioeconomic circumstances in eighteenth-century Vienna. It is well known that Mozart had prodigious gifts as a musician; he could sing, and play the piano and the violin flawlessly; he could improvise on themes that he had just heard and at a very early age he began to compose. Yet Mozart went beyond these gifts to develop a musical voice uniquely his own, which continues profoundly to engage and touch listeners today. We are awed by the prodigy and moved by the creative genius.

What made it possible for this boy, dominated by his father and dragged at an early age from provincial capitals to great cities, to perform his precocious miracles, to become a mature explorer of the human condition? How did his family, his health, his musical education, his own inner conflicts contribute to the artist that he was to become? How did his precociousness both aid and hinder his creative vitality? And what do Mozart's experiences contribute to our greater knowledge of that mysterious passage from prodigy to genius? Those were some of the questions we set out to explore.

Our contributors are a diverse group of experts; they are psychologists, child psychotherapists, physicians, musicologists, historians, and performing artists. All have obviously been touched by Mozart and wish to understand his genius without simply explaining it away. None pretended to have all the answers. Perhaps this task is like the music of the man himself. He was immersed in the forms and musical devices of his day but he filled the conventions that he found with something transcendent and yet beautifully earthy.

The book begins with an informative analysis, by one of the world's leading experts in this field, of how genius is recognized and defined. Professor Dean Keith Simonton has done extensive historiometric research, and while he modestly disclaims any special expertise on Mozart it soon becomes apparent that the statistical analysis of the large cohort of geniuses he has assembled can result in substantial correlations between creative originality and such factors as age, life events, and emotional orientation. Thus one arrives at a profile of genius that may have predictive validity and should be an excellent guide for the teacher, praticing therapist, or parent concerned with problems of an especially gifted child.

The next chapter, by Professor David Henry Feldman, deals with the child prodigy, potentially a precursor to genius, and thus moves a little closer to Mozart specifically. Dr. Feldman has closely observed the personality development of prodigious individuals and addresses their characteristic family environments, patterns of upbringing, character traits, emotional crises, and accomplishments. His contributions are relevant to the task of providing unusual children with appropriate educational opportunities that are conducive not only to continuing excellence but, it is hoped, to a successful life as well.

Erna Schwerin's chapter leads directly to Wolfgang Amadeus Mozart, that extraordinary boy growing up in a musical family dominated by his father, with an older sister who is herself a promising musician, and a mother who must make sure that all of them get enough food, sleep, proper clothing, and other necessities of life. With her extensive experience as a psychotherapist, Schwerin, who is also an outstanding Mozart scholar, presents the human side of genius: how the members of this unusual family related to each other, resulting inevitably in much joy and many frustrations.

Unfortunately some of the most important components of the conference that led to this book cannot be reproduced. These consisted of musical performances and spontaneous, informal discussions. For example, Erna Schwerin's paper about the Mozart family

was followed by a performance and commentary on the childhood
pieces written by Mozart. First came compositions for piano alone,
written in a barely legible child's hand with generous assistance from
Papa Mozart. These were played by Jonathan Khuner, a pianist and
conductor then with the San Francisco Opera and now with the new
Tel Aviv Opera Company in Israel. He was joined at the keyboard
by violinist Dr. Peter Ostwald for a performance of Mozart's earliest
piano-violin sonatas, demonstrating the lingering influence of his father (a violinist who played these works with Wolfgang), as well as the
integration into his own music of musical styles to which the traveling
child prodigy was progressively exposed while on tour through Austria, Germany, France, England, and Italy. Mr. Khuner commented
on each of the pieces played and also performed compositions by
Johann Schobert, Johann Christian Bach, Carl Friedrich Abel, and
Leopold Mozart himself, all prominent eighteenth-century composers
who influenced the child Mozart. Mr. Khuner was then joined at the
keyboard by Lise Deschamps Ostwald for a performance of Mozart's
early four-handed piano works (played originally with his sister Nannerl). Finally some of Mozart's very first orchestral writings were performed, again showing the marvellous combination of innate originality and adherence to standards expected within the musical culture
of Europe in the last eighteenth century.

Dr. Leonard Zegans's paper is about secular awe and our fascination with the genius phenomenon, which cannot be separated from
present-day concerns about survival and the meaning of life. It includes a brilliantly invented letter from Mozart to his father, illustrat-
ing certain of the themes touched on in other chapters in this book.
This is followed by Dr. Gary Gelber's exploration of the ways in which
Mozart expressed his divergent self-images, particularly the striking
contrast between his outward cockiness and inwardly low self-esteem.
Much (too much, considering the ill-chosen diagnosis of Gilles de la
Tourette's disease recently proposed for Mozart) has been made
about the composer's scatological humor, discussed here from a psychodynamic perspective.

The next two chapters are concerned with medical aspects, first
the general situation of clinical practice when Mozart lived in Vienna,
then the specific questions that have arisen concerning Mozart's illnesses, treatment, and death. Dr. Günter Risse depicts the precarious
health conditions in the Habsburg Empire at that time, including a
population explosion, widespread nutritional deficiencies, a very high

rate of infant mortality, and epidemics of infectious diseases. This historical survey cannot help but highlight the remarkable progress that has been made since Mozart's time in general hygiene, hospital care, medical education, and therapeutics, and this emphasizes the health risks facing a musician like Mozart. These risks are addressed directly in the chapter by Dr. Peter Davies, who discusses how Mozart survived an incredible array of serious infections such as typhoid fever, smallpox, and hepatitis. The composer also suffered from a number of chronic diseases, mostly infectious and immunological reactions. Dr. Davies reviews the controversies about Mozart's skull, circumstances surrounding his terminal illness, and his pitiful death at age 35.

Certain developments in the life of the genius Mozart as he matured are presented next. First we hear from concert pianist Paul Hersh, whose chapter begins with an appreciation of Mozart as performer. Again, this part of the conference featured live performances (by Mr. Hersh) that cannot be reproduced in the book. What makes Mozart's music so especially appealing, moving, and captivating is explored in the second part of his chapter, illustrated with musical examples that show how by changing just a few notes Mozart's music loses its characteristic mixture of sadness and happiness and starts sounding rather ordinary.

Dr. Stuart Feder expands on this subject by bringing his combined psychoanalytic and musicological skills to bear on the question of Mozart's compositions in D minor. These works often seem to allude quite directly to certain problems in the composer's life, his family relationships, and especially the struggle with his father over autonomy. The father's "curse" is heard to echo in a number of Mozart's greatest compositions. Professor Thomas Bauman goes further into this topic with a brilliant analysis of the three trials of Don Giovanni. Each trial adheres to a common paradigm: A misdeed of the "young, licentious nobleman" leads to a confrontation in the form of the trial mechanism sanctioned by cultural practice for the offense in question. Bauman's cultural analysis of themes surrounding male sexual aggression is pertinent to contemporary psychotherapeutic issues.

The startling fact that Mozart left a long trail of unfinished compositions is discussed by Professor Robert Marshall, who during his talk demonstrated a number of these fragmentary works. They reflect fluctuating circumstances of Mozart's life and shed light on changes in his working methods during the course of his career. One of the most controversial unfinished works is the famous *Requiem*, Mozart's final composition, and Dr. George Pollock's chapter describes the need to correct various myths that have grown up around this composition as well as around other aspects of Mozart's life. Recent scholarly criticism is reviewed, and Pollock concludes that many of the mysteries about him may never be solved.

Dr. Ostwald's chapter begins with a historical review of the genius/madness controversy and describes changing views related to religious beliefs, the influence of the Renaissance, positive attitudes developed during the era of enlightenment, the haunting vision of romanticism, and the scientific era with its shift from neurodegenerative to psychoanalytic theories. A case example, that of the dancer Vaslav Nijinsky, is given to illustrate the contrast between healthy and pathological behavior in the life of a genius. Which direction an individual life will go, whether toward genius or toward mental disorder or even toward both, seems to depend on critical moments in development whose outcome remains largely unpredictable.

The book closes with a panel of eminent Mozart performers—a singer, a violinist, an opera director, and two pianists—talking about their personal experience as childhood musicians and how that experience has affected their adult careers generally and their interpretation of Mozart's music specifically.

During the discussions that followed these papers and the informal conversations after the scheduled sessions, there was a palpable sense of the deep affection people have for Mozart's music and their gratitude for the ways in which it has enhanced their lives. We discussed some puzzling contradictions in Mozart's immense originality, his marked dependency, his great stamina, his tragic poor health, his *joie de vivre*, his financial despair, in short both the pleasures and the perils of a short but immensely productive life without simply reducing him to a "case." Inspired by his universality, the speakers discovered a common love for Mozart's music expressing simplicity, complexity, and humanity. We hope that some of the feelings stimulated by this symposium will come through to readers of the published papers and transcend the task of just explaining Mozart.

A number of persons and organizations contributed significantly to the success of the symposium this book is based on, and we wish to acknowledge their substantial assistance: Chancellor and Mrs. Julius Krevans of the University of California in San Francisco; Sara Burke,

Director of UCSF's Extended Programs in Medical Education; Samuel H. Barondes, M.D., Chairman of the Department of Psychiatry; Nina Beckwith, Administrative Director of UCSF's Health Program for Performing Artists; the Friends of Langley Porter, the Goethe Institute, and the "Café Mozart" in San Francisco. We are grateful to Martin Azarian and the staff of International Universities Press for helping us transform the symposium into a book.

REFERENCE

Rothstein, E. (1991), "Mozart's bicentennial: Too much, too late." *New York Times*, Sec. 2, December 1, pp. 31–32.

1

Creative Genius in Music: Mozart and Other Composers

Dean Keith Simonton, Ph.D.

Let this chapter begin with a confession: Unlike some of the other authors in this volume, I am by no means an expert on Mozart. While I am a music lover, I cannot even claim that Mozart is my favorite composer—albeit to my tastes he does join in an unchallenged triumvirate with Beethoven and Bach. Thus, my qualifications for contributing an essay on Mozart must come from another quarter; namely, that I have devoted well over a hundred publications to the scientific study of historical genius in virtually all domains of enduring achievement. Some of my studies have focused on genius in leadership activities, such as politics and war, while other studies have focused on creative disciplines, such as science and art (Simonton, 1984b). Almost all of these inquiries exploit "historiometric" techniques. That is, large computer data bases are compiled on hundreds if not thousands of exemplars of a particular type of genius, and the resulting information is subjected to comprehensive and precise analysis, using either multivariate statistics or mathematical models (Simonton, 1990b). This approach is designed to tease out the broad patterns in the lives and careers of many geniuses—probabilistic regularities that help us create an abstract profile of the typical genius in a given area of eminence. We are obviously not dealing here with a fine-grained procedure dedicated to explicating the minutiae regarding individual creators or leaders, but rather historiometry is limited to defining the generic qualities manifested by most geniuses of a given type.

Needless to say, that I can call upon some expertise regarding the attributes of genius still does not necessarily qualify me to write on Mozart. Genius though he was, his contribution was restricted to music. Even so, a significant portion of my research program has focused on musical genius in the classical repertoire. Typically I have investigated the lives and works of anywhere between ten and 696 classical composers (e.g., Simonton, 1977a, 1991a,b); just once I did allot a whole investigation to the compositions of a single composer, and that lone exception concerned Beethoven (Simonton, 1987b). Using the compiled data bases, the characteristics of musical genius are scrutinized from a diversity of perspectives, each often requiring a distinct unit of analysis. While sometimes the analytical unit is the composer, other times the cases shift to separate musical themes, individual compositions, or consecutive five-year periods in a composer's life. Moreover, on occasion the inquiries concentrate on the biographical circumstances of musical creativity, whereas more often the concentration resides with the aesthetic attributes of the works produced.

Whatever the specifics, this body of research should allow me to venture at least a few remarks concerning the generic profile of the musical genius. This liberty receives all the more endorsement by the fact that, with the sole exception of the Beethoven case study, Mozart was not excluded from any inquiry. Indeed, in those studies that employed the theme or composition as the analytical unit, Mozart's example was quite conspicuous. For instance, in a content analysis of 5046 themes by ten classical composers (Simonton, 1980a), Mozart contributed fully 833 melodies, or 17 percent of the total melodic material—more than Bach or Beethoven or anyone else. Consequently, Mozart's genius perforce provided a major input in constructing the final profile, leading us to suspect that he must be to some reasonable extent quite representative of the generic portrait. The outcome of the Beethoven case study should strengthen our confidence in this congruence, for one aim of that investigation was to show that Beethoven's musical career fit the pattern already established for the entire set of composers whose masterworks appear in the standard repertoire (Simonton, 1987b). Naturally, no individual will comply with every minute feature of an abstract profile, no more than we can easily identify perfect exemplars of the diverse clinical diagnostic categories. Nonetheless, by delineating the common characteristics of the musical genius, we can raise a backdrop that enables us to comprehend more fully the distinctiveness of a Mozart.

Now that the method of attack has been outlined, we can turn to the problem of defining what we mean by *genius*, with emphasis on how we can justify assigning that label to Mozart. After completing that more analytical task, we can review the key empirical findings about musical genius. At various points along the way we will discuss how or whether Mozart exemplifies the emerging picture, a topic that will be developed further in this chapter's coda as well.

DEFINITION OF GENIUS

The term *genius* has a very long history (Murray, 1989). Etymologically, it dates back to Roman times, when each individual had a guiding spirit that helped determine a person's uniqueness and destiny. In a sense, the genius was the "generator" of an individual's personality. By the time the Romantics expropriated the word, it had acquired far more momentous implications: Only a few people could claim true "genius," namely those celebrities who managed to make some extraordinary contribution to human civilization—by some accomplishment so distinctive and so powerful that history was necessarily transformed. Hence, the term was reserved for the likes of Napoleon, Newton, Descartes, Shakespeare, Michelangelo, and, yes, Mozart. Fortunately, more objective, even quantifiable definitions are available, usages that permit a more scientific view of the phenomenon. In particular, the behavioral scientist now has two options, the psychometric and the historiometric.

PSYCHOMETRIC GENIUS

Near the beginning of this century, Alfred Binet devised the first successful measure of intelligence, an instrument that eventually evolved into the much abused "IQ test." An important figure in this evolution was Lewis Terman who, in a series of volumes collectively entitled *Genetic Studies of Genius*, presented results of one of the most ambitious longitudinal studies in the history of the behavioral sciences (e.g., Terman, 1925; Terman and Oden, 1959). Significantly, Terman's operational definition of genius was a score on the Stanford-Binet of around three standard deviations above the mean—or about IQ 145. While we can certainly debate the best IQ cutoff for assigning the genius label, the point should not be missed that Terman's approach had the virtue of providing an objective procedure for identifying geniuses, one that has been widely followed in the literature on gifted children ever since (see also Hollingworth, 1926). Even today, and especially in the popular press, someone who scores exceptionally high on an IQ test is automatically styled a "genius." (The MENSA society is a club of self-styled geniuses who score at least two standard deviations above the mean in psychometric intelligence.)

It would seem that this definition gets us nowhere if we wish to address whether Mozart counts as a genius. After all, he died over a century before IQ tests were available. But a route exists around this difficulty. Terman (1917) showed how IQ scores could be estimated from sufficiently detailed biographical materials about the early childhood and adolescence of any historical figure. This application is founded on the idea that IQ is defined as a person's mental age divided by chronological age (multiplied by 100), thus getting the "intelligence quotient." As an illustration, Terman (1917) carefully inspected the early years of Francis Galton, a decidedly precocious genius, and arrived at an estimate close to IQ 200. Thus, when Galton was around 5, he had the intellectual wherewithal of a 10-year-old. Happily, one of Terman's graduate students, Catherine Cox (1926), extended this procedure to 301 creators and leaders of European civilization, providing us with priceless IQ scores.

It goes without saying that Mozart was among those for whom an IQ was estimated. As Cox (1926) and her research assistants saw it, Mozart's score was between 150 and 155 (or between 160 and 165 once corrected for data reliability). These estimates are comfortably past the usual threshold for designating someone a psychometric genius. Furthermore, of the ten other composers assigned IQs in this study, only Mendelssohn matched Mozart's estimate, and not one exceeded him. For instance, Beethoven's estimates ranged between 135 and 140, and Bach's were lower still. Clearly, largely because Mozart was one of the most precocious composers of all time, he qualified as one of the brightest as well. Of course, many criticisms can be made regarding these estimates—far too many to list here—but at least if we take Terman's (1917) method and Cox's (1926) calculations at face value, there can be little doubt that Mozart satisfied the psychometric criterion for genius.

HISTORIOMETRIC GENIUS

A common complaint with the psychometric definition of genius is that there is little relationship between IQ and success in almost any human endeavor (McClelland, 1973). For instance, eminent scientists, even those winning Nobel prizes, cannot boast higher scores than their far less illustrious colleagues (Simonton, 1988c). Indeed, the individual with the highest IQ on record, Marilyn Vos Savant (IQ 230), has yet to impress anyone with a single outstanding accomplishment—other than making it into the *Guinness Book of Records* and writing a column in which she gives smart answers to dumb questions. Therefore, even if we accept Cox's (1926) IQ estimates, we must be wary about using them to draw any grand inferences. Certainly it would be unwise to maintain that because Mozart's IQ was about one standard deviation higher than Beethoven's, the former is the better composer (but see Simonton, 1991b). Hence, we might be better advised to lean on a scientific definition of genius that is more intimately related to actual accomplishment. Interestingly, back in 1869 just such a concept was offered by the supremely brilliant Francis Galton. In his classic book *Hereditary Genius*, Galton conceived of genius in terms of posthumous reputation or eminence. This operational definition is still vague until it is translated into more specific terms, which can be done in two principal ways (Simonton, 1990b).

First, we can ask the experts to offer us their opinions. In the specific case of classical music, for example, we can survey musicologists, asking them to rate the diverse contributors to the repertoire. Farnsworth (1969) conducted just such an inquiry, obtaining evaluations of all-time eminence from respondents who were members of the American Musicological Society. The top ten composers were, in order, J. S. Bach, Beethoven, Mozart, Haydn, Brahms, Handel, Debussy, Schubert, Wagner, and Chopin. One may quibble with this list until doomsday—especially if one's favorite composer is farther down the ordinal sequence—yet I think it safe to conclude that Mozart's posthumous reputation is among the best. It is difficult to conceive of anyone below him, out of the 100 ranked, who would deserve a higher place.

Second, and perhaps most pertinent, we can gauge more directly the impact that a given historical personality has had on subsequent generations. In the instance of classical music, such an assessment becomes especially convenient; rather than survey a sample of experts, we can more simply determine how frequently various composers are performed and recorded—in other words, whose creations dominate the repertoire. To illustrate, Moles (1958) tabulated the relative performance frequencies of work by 250 classical composers. The top ten on this list are Mozart (6.1%), Beethoven (5.9%), J. S. Bach (5.9%), Wagner (4.2%), Brahms (4.1%), Schubert (3.6%), Handel (2.8%), Tchaikovsky (2.8%), Verdi (2.5%), and Haydn (2.3%). Although composers popular with audiences are not identical with those respected by musicologists, the overall picture is not radically different, especially when the two rival lists are closely compared. As a case in point, Tartini ends up in the 100th place in both rankings (and the correlation between the two assessments is .72). Most critical for current discussion, Mozart is a clear favorite with those who have to pay for the admission tickets. By this second criterion, without question, Mozart makes the grade as a first-rate musical genius.

Other methods exist, naturally, for tapping an individual's posthumous reputation—such as frequency of recordings, inclusion in music appreciation textbooks and anthologies, the amount of space granted in music encyclopedias, histories, and biographical dictionaries—but it really does not make much difference anyhow. Sophisticated psychometric analyses of alternative eminence measures show quite conclusively that a tremendous consensus exists on the relative merits of the composers who define the classical repertoire; furthermore, this consensus is extremely stable over considerable periods of time (Farnsworth, 1969; Simonton, 1991c). The last point bears special emphasis, given how fickle fashion is so often thought to be. The ups and downs of taste are minuscule in comparison to the awesome inertia of true merit. How often in the history of music, for instance, has Schenk or Pleyel surpassed Mozart in esteem? So Mozart's place in the annals of musical genius is solid.

THE LIFE OF GENIUS

The historiometric gauge of genius is the one favored in all of my own inquiries into musical creativity. Besides yielding highly reliable indicators of eminence, such measures enjoy a face validity not found in any alternative; the average connoisseur believes that Mozart was a greater composer than Salieri not because Mozart had a higher IQ but rather because Mozart produced a far larger body of compositions that cannot be lived without. In any case, using this operational definition, we can inquire into those characteristics that are most strongly associated with an individual's being able to climb to the Olympian heights. We begin with an examination of the early developmental experiences that may contribute to the later attainment of greatness and then turn to a survey of the chief features of a creative career in music composition.

DEVELOPMENTAL ANTECEDENTS

A large literature has accumulated on the conditions and events in childhood and adolescence that enhance the odds that an individual will achieve distinction in adulthood (Simonton, 1987a). Some of these developmental experiences are germane to all forms of achievement, others are confined to particular domains of genius. All operate in a probabilistic fashion rather than being deterministic in impact, and accordingly numerous exceptions exist to any given statistical association. This limitation should be kept in mind, for it implies that we certainly cannot expect Mozart to fit the developmental profile on every count. Strictly speaking, the probability of total compliance for any single genius is for all practical purposes zero. In any case, let us briefly examine the following five developmental factors:

    1. *Birth Order*. Francis Galton (1874) was the first behavioral scientist to observe that first-born children, and especially first-born sons, are disproportionately represented among the eminent, a finding replicated often over the past century (see also Ellis, 1904). Even if artistic and revolutionary genius tends to depart from this pattern (Bliss, 1970; Stewart, 1977), the supremacy of the first-born son has been shown to hold for classical composers as well (Schubert, Wagner, and Schubert, 1977). In fact, in this respect, classical composers are more akin to scientists than artists in other media of aesthetic expression (Simonton, 1988c). Mozart at first seems an exception to this tendency insofar as he was the seventh and last child. Yet most of his older siblings died in infancy, and the sibling closest to him in age, Nannerl, was both female and five years older. Furthermore, in many ways Wolfgang's father, Leopold, treated his last born as if he were a first born, showing a tremendous interest in his son's musical and intellectual development. Because it has been frequently argued that

the chief advantage of the first born is the special attention they tend to receive from parents (Albert, 1980), Mozart may not mark such a discrepancy after all.

2. *Orphanhood.* Geniuses in virtually every domain of achievement, whether entailing creativity or leadership, appear to suffer high rates of emotional trauma, especially parental loss, in childhood and adolescence (Eisenstadt, 1978). The occurrence of such adverse experiences is notably conspicuous in the lives of artistic creators, such as poets, and somewhat less evident in scientific creators, such as physicists (Simonton, 1988c). Because Mozart's mother died when he was 22, and his father when he was 29, he may be said to contradict this pattern. Nonetheless, to the extent that classical composition has greater creative affinities with doing science than art—in their shared dependence on highly abstract forms of expression governed by mathematical rules—this contrast may not be all that critical anyway. It can be speculated, however, that the losses of his mother and father in early adulthood may have played no small role in encouraging Mozart to deepen his style, introducing that profound melancholy that so often permeates the masterworks in the last half decade of his life. Indirect evidence for this possiblity will come later in this essay.

3. *Family Pedigree.* It was Galton's (1869) goal in his *Hereditary Genius* to show that geniuses in all walks of life tend to be concentrated in family lines of distinguished figures in the same achievement domain. In his chapter on composers, he offers the family tree of Johann Sebastian Bach as a supreme example of this tendency. All told, there were at least two dozen musically distinguished Bachs, whether ancestors or progeny, and four of J. S. Bach's own sons attained considerable distinction, one even temporarily eclipsing his father's renown. Galton also includes the Mozart family in his compilations and tabulations, albeit here the family pedigree is not nearly so preeminent. Wolfgang's father, Leopold, was not without merit as a composer, and had written an influential treatise on violin playing; Wolfgang's sister, Nannerl, displayed some glimmer of talent, although she was hardly in the same class as her younger brother (nor was she in the same league as Fanny Mendelssohn); and Wolfgang had a posthumous son, Wolfgang the Younger, who managed to compose some competent music, but certainly without coming anywhere near matching the creativity of his greater contemporaries, such as Schubert. That's it! Even so, we should not disparage Mozart's musical pedigree too much, for at least he surpassed Beethoven on this criterion. And

the likelihood that Mozart would have any eminent relatives at all by chance alone remains incredibly tiny.

4. *Role Models.* Notwithstanding the theoretical impetus behind Galton's (1869) studies, it is still unclear why geniuses are so often embedded in family pedigrees. While Galton himself thought he had established a genetic foundation for outstanding achievement, according to modern studies in behavioral genetics the jury is still out (Simonton, 1983b). Many critics have argued that environmental factors may deserve the lion's share of credit for any familial connections (Simonton, 1987a). In particular, the appearance of family pedigrees may be nothing more than a special case of the far more general finding that notable figures tend to have access, often very early in life, to individuals who provide models of achievement in the domain where distinction is eventually attained (e.g., Simonton, 1975, 1983b, 1984a, 1988b). These models may be admired and emulated at a distance, or may assume a more active role as mentors or teachers. There is no reason to doubt that this social-learning process occurs in classical music (Simonton, 1977b), nor is Mozart in any manner an exception to this rule. Besides the mentorship of his father, Mozart was very early in life exposed to the musical ideas of Johann Christian Bach, distinguished son of J. S. Bach and a family friend. In addition, the young Mozart grew up in the midst of a rich musical tradition of instrumental, vocal, and dramatic composition, a tradition in which he could encounter and assimilate, whether directly or indirectly, the creativity of many other composers ranging from the now obscure Schobert to the still distinguished Franz Joseph Haydn. On this score, Mozart's fit with the typical profile is snug indeed.

5. *Expertise Acquisition.* Contrary to widespread myths, genius does not emerge suddenly out of thin air like Athena from the head of Zeus. Rather, it generally requires, on the average, a good decade of learning and practice to master any discipline before one can expect to make a truly original contribution, a constraint that has been shown to hold in the specific case of classical music as well (Hayes, 1989, pp. 293–299). To be sure, Mozart seems to be an exception, given how quickly the young child prodigy began to compose after Leopold began Wolfgang's musical training. Nevertheless, we must observe that Mozart's early pieces did not show any particular merit; to paraphrase Samuel Johnson's critique of a dog walking on his hind legs, it was not so much that he did it well but that he did it at all. His first genuine masterpieces, judging by what made it into the standard

repertoire, did not appear until his late teens, easily ten full years after his compositional labors commenced (Hayes, 1989). Incidentally, this fifth developmental factor links with the preceding one, for there is evidence that the more role models are available for emulation, the earlier training begins, and hence the more precocious the creative output (Simonton, 1977b). Born at the right place at the right time, Mozart was all set to become one of the greatest musical prodigies of all time (see also Feldman, 1986).

CAREER PERFORMANCE

Once a creative career takes off, it tends to pursue an identifiable trajectory over the life span (Simonton, 1988a). In the case of the classical repertoire, in particular, the "average musical genius" begins composition around the late teens, produces his first unqualified masterwork in the late twenties, output thereafter accelerating until a peak is reached in the late thirties, at which time his best compositions tend to appear, after which productivity tends gradually to decline, the final masterpiece emerging in the early fifties, the composer then dying somewhere in his middle sixties (Simonton, 1991b). This general career trajectory can be deflected by extraneous events, such as war and physical illness, but the departures are prone to be transient rather than permanent (Simonton, 1977a). However, the typical trajectory does vary significantly according to the amount of genius exhibited—a critical consideration given our interest in determining how Mozart fits with the profile. Specifically, the more impressive the accomplishment, the earlier composition begins, the sooner the first "hit," and the later the last "hit," whereas the age of peak output and best works as well as the age at death are not contingent upon the magnitude of achievement (Simonton, 1991b). Looking at Mozart, it is obvious that he initiated his career corresponding to the pattern typical for genuine luminaries: He was approximately a decade precocious regarding both the commencement of his compositional endeavors and the creation of his first masterwork. On the other hand, owing to the fact that he died young, his career was not allowed to play out the remainder of the pattern. Mozart died in his thirty-sixth year, this when the life expectancy for composers in his day was 63 (Simonton, 1977b). Nonetheless, as he was still going strong in his last year—producing compositions of the caliber of the *Requiem* and *The Magic*

Flute—we can quite reasonably conjecture that he had not yet peaked, and would have had a long and productive career ahead.

Ironically, it was Mozart's very extreme precocity that enabled him to die so young—only Schubert and Pergolesi among notable composers died younger—and still make it into the annals of music. Empirical inquiries into genius consistently show that an early career onset is associated with an early death (Simonton, 1977b, 1991a). It is not so much a matter that the extremely precocious burn themselves out early as a simple fact that only by producing masterpieces at a youthful age can one die young and still earn a place in posterity. Had Bruckner died as young as Mozart, it is most unlikely that his name would be known at all today.

Although a tragic early death prevented Mozart from realizing the final portion of the anticipated career trajectory, this event miraculously did not deny him the capacity to exhibit another striking feature of exceptional creative careers—unusual lifetime productivity (Simonton, 1984b). In most domains of human achievement, a small proportion of participating individuals account for the bulk of all contributions. Typically the achievers who constitute the top 10 percent in lifetime output are responsible for around 50 percent of everything produced, whereas the individuals who are below the fiftieth percentile in total productivity can be credited with only about 15 percent of the entire collection of contributions; moreover, the distribution of output is so skewed right that the modal score is a single contribution, from which point the frequencies monotonically decline as the lifetime productivity count increases (Dennis, 1955). Of course, this highly elitist distribution is implicit in the relative performance frequencies tabulated by Moles (1958), for the top three composers account for 18 percent of all works heard. The Moles data also illustrate the Price law which is sometimes used to describe the disparity between the prolific few and the nearly silent many (Simonton, 1984b, 1988c). According to this law, if k is taken to represent the number of persons who have contributed something of value to a given field, then the square root of this number (i.e., $\sqrt{k}$) approximates the number of individuals whose names can be identified with half of the whole. Since Moles found that roughly 250 composers are responsible for at least one work in the classical repertoire, the square root of this number is 15.8. This prediction is remarkably close to Moles's indication that sixteen composers account for half of all compositions regularly performed and recorded! And, needless to say, Mozart stands at the apex of this elite as the cream of the cream.

One complication lurks in the previous paragraph, namely the distinction between quantity and quality of output. Does it make a difference whether we scrutinize total output, ignoring aesthetic success, or confine our analysis to that subset of pieces that have had an actual impact on colleagues or connoisseurs? The answer is, simply, no. To be sure, there occasionally emerge perfectionists who produce only a handful of works, and all these of extremely high quality. And there do appear from time to time mass producers who generate at a hectic pace without conceiving a single noteworthy creation. But perfectionists and mass producers are exceptions to the general scheme of things. For the most part, quality is positively associated with quality, so that those creators who produce the most memorable works also then, on the average, produce the most forgettable works (Simonton, 1984b). Moreover, a creator's success rate does not systematically alter over the course of a career; no matter how mature the individual, the proportion of hits to total attempts stays roughly constant across the life span (Simonton, 1988a). Anyone with considerable familiarity with the over 600 works that have been assigned Köchel numbers would have no problem concluding that Mozart marks no departure from this statistical regularity. When I was a graduate student at Harvard, the campus radio station once put on a Mozart marathon, playing almost every piece by that composer in strict chronological order. What I experienced was a random mix of sublime music marked by Mozart's magical gift side by side with utterly pedestrian hackwork and experimental rejects. A detailed analysis of the careers of the top ten composers in Farnsworth's (1969) survey demonstrated that this haphazard production of the good and the bad is characteristic of all great composers (Simonton, 1977a).

THE WORKS OF GENIUS

We have just learned that not every composition by a Mozart is a masterpiece, and that the output of most creators is typically uneven in quality. And yet there is ample evidence that a creator's reputation is predicated on producing a respectable number of works that posterity can designate as masterpieces (Albert, 1975; Simonton, 1991c). This leads us to shift our attention from matters of creativity to issues of aesthetics, requiring us to alter our unit of analysis from the composer to the composition. Here I will survey the key results of a research program based on a principle that on first glance might appear completely preposterous—the *computerized* content analysis of the thematic material that makes up the classical repertoire. Although every reader has the right to be skeptical, the procedure has been tested and validated so many times and in so many ways, that I cannot help but believe that the findings contribute to our understanding of musical genius (Simonton, 1983a). But first, we need a little background and justification.

Paisley (1964) was among the first to show how much a dumb computer can glean from the most minimal information about a musical composition. Intrigued by whether a computer can be programmed to identify the creator of a musical piece, he began with a large sample of themes from several classical composers, including Bach, Beethoven, and, yes, Mozart. Only the first four notes were used, and each theme was transposed to a C tonic (i.e., either C major or C minor). Instrumentation, rhythm, counterpoint, and a host of other parameters were essentially obliterated, granting the computer only the consecutive notes. Then the computer calculated the two-note transition probabilities in order to discern the characteristic routes by which each composer constructed his melodies. For example, what are the odds that a composer will go from the dominant to the subdominant versus the dominant to the tonic? Who most often employs chromatic transitions? Which composer most frequently repeats notes? (The answer, among those examined, is Mozart!) Once these stylistic proclivities were estimated for each composer, the computer was given a batch of test melodies that were not contained in the sets from which the transition probabilities were originally tabulated. On this basis, the computer would determine the odds that a test batch was created by each of the various composers studied. The actual composer of the test melodies almost invariably turned out to be the individual whom the computer picked out as having the highest likelihood of creating those themes! That a computer could do so well—even better than many a hapless student in a music appreciation course—led me to ask if the computer can discern more than just a composer's style?

To find out, I took all those themes contained in a two-volume thematic dictionary (Barlow and Morgenstern, 1948, 1976), deleting only those which failed to satisfy certain a priori criteria, yielding

15,618 themes by 479 classical composers—virtually every piece in the classical repertoire as of the middle of this century (Simonton, 1980b). To be on the safe side, the first *six* notes were investigated for each theme, but othewise the same procedure was followed as developed by Paisley (1964). In particular, the two-note transition probabilities were estimated across the entire set of themes. It became quite clear that some transitions are extremely commonplace, whereas others are rather rare. For example, merely going from G to G (i.e., repeating the dominant) occurs in almost 7 percent of all transitions, a popularity that surpasses even the C-C (i.e., tonic repetition) transition, which stands at a bit over 5 percent. In contrast, chromatic transitions, which includes all sharps and flats except the three in the C Minor scale (E flat, B flat, and A flat), are found in fewer than 1 percent of all themes (see Simonton, 1984c).

Given these probabilities for all possible two-note transitions, the computer was then programmed to calculate for each theme an attribute styled *melodic originality*, which is essentially a gauge of how improbable a given string of six notes is in the context of the entire classical repertoire (correcting, by the by, for the number of themes each composer contributed to that repertoire). For instance, the initial theme to the second movement of Haydn's Surprise Symphony starts C-C-E-E-G-G, yielding a mundane melody that sounds an awful lot like "Twinkle, Twinkle, Little Star." In contrast, one of the quartets Mozart dedicated to Haydn (K. 465) has an introduction which begins A-G-F#-G-A-B flat, producing an effect so striking that the piece earned the name "The Dissonant." When Haydn was asked what he thought of the passage, he could only respond "If Mozart composed it, he must have had a reason!" It enhances our confidence in the computer's judgment that it decided the Haydn theme had a probability of appearing in the classical repertoire that was four times higher than that of Mozart's.

At this juncture it may behoove us to counter potential skepticism about whether such an objective, computerized calculation has any bearing whatsoever on real music experience. After all, the measure is admittedly crude, built as it is on only the first six notes, and even then ignoring all aspects of a theme except how the notes of a scale pass from one to the next. Fortunately, a series of validation studies make a convincing case that the computer has actually identified something of aesthetic significance (Simonton, 1990b, pp. 113–118). May a few instances suffice.

1. When naive listeners hear tape recordings of the melody line played on a violin and judge these simplified stimuli according to "arousal potential," the resulting ratings correlate respectably with the objective indicators of originality (Martindale and Uemura, 1983). In addition, using the first six notes, we can do an even better job than Paisley (1964) did in identifying the style of hundreds of composers, stylistic contrasts that are intuitively experienced by persons well versed in the repertoire (Simonton, 1980b, 1986).

2. Melodic originality derived from two-note transition probabilities correlate extremely high with those derived from three-note probabilities (Simonton, 1980a, 1984c). Consequently, the calculations do not depend on the specific means by which we estimate a theme's predictability.

3. The computer's assessments correspond with other facets of a musical composition in a sensible manner. For instance, melodic originality is higher for themes written in a minor key relative to those in a major key (Simonton, 1987b), a finding in keeping with the more exotic flavor of minor-key melodies. Melodic originality is more prominent in instrumental works than in vocal music, a fact reflecting both the technical constraints on the human voice as well as the need to prevent the melody from overpowering the text (Simonton, 1980b). In a similar vein, melodic originality tends to be high in chamber music, such as sonatas and quartets, medium in orchestral music, such as symphonies, tone poems, and overtures, and low in theater music, such as opera and ballet (Simonton, 1980b). If one takes an information-processing perspective (Moles, 1958), and assumes that the total cognitive demand imposed by a piece is a function of all the stimulatory forces available to the composer, then clearly chamber works are going to require melodic content to carry most of the load, whereas theatrical works can allow many other auditory, visual, and semantic channels to share the labors.

4. The level of melodic originality displayed by a composer's compositions in part depends on the larger biographical context of the creator's career. One case in point is the inverse relationship between melodic originality and a composer's concomitant level of thematic productivity (Simonton, 1986). Those years when a composer tends to generate melodies at a hectic pace tend to be the same years when their less profound melodies appear, indicating something of a tradeoff between quantity and quality in this restricted situation

(Simonton, 1977a). At an even more comprehensive level, the intensity of level of melodic originality favored by a particular composer is contingent, at least in part, on that composer's geographic marginality. This circumstance was defined as the physical distance between the place where the composer was born and those locations that can be taken as the centers of music activity for the day (for details see Simonton [1977b]). Hence, those who were born and raised far away may be considered "provincials," those at or near the centers "cosmopolitans." In any case, the more proximate a composer to the hot spots of musical creativity, the higher the expected level of his or her melodic originality (Simonton, 1986). The core areas very likely place a greater premium on innovation and novelty in comparison to the more restraining conventions of the provinces. Provincials are even less prolific in thematic output than are cosmopolitans (Simonton, 1977b).

5. Melodic originality varies across historical time as well as over the surface of the globe: If scores for the 15,618 themes are plotted as a function of the theme's composition date, and then a trend line fitted to the resulting scatterplot, we obtain a description of how this aesthetic attribute has tended to fluctuate over the course of the Western musical tradition (Simonton, 1980b). According to this trend analysis (which yields a fifth-order polynomial function), melodic originality starts at its lowest level around 1500, as is evident from listening to Renaissance dances or the masses of Josquin des Pres. But from that low point melodic originality climbed rather quickly to a peak in the early Baroque, as represented most daringly in the motets of Monteverdi and Gesualdo. The latter's "Moro lasso," for example, begins G#-G-F#-F-F-B, a sequence consisting of transitions that are extremely rare in the classical repertoire. After this ascent leveled off around 1650, a decline commenced, as composers found other ways to heighten a composition's interest, including elaborate counterpoint, more complex forms, and richer instrumentation. Melodic originality accordingly reached a secondary low just before 1800—the period of the classical period epitomized by Haydn, Mozart, and early Beethoven. In this era, melodies were often constructed around simple chords, even triads, as the primary focus centered on developing germinal ideas via such forms as the sonata-allegro. Melodic originality in this period was about half way between that of the Renaissance and that of the early Baroque. But starting in the nineteenth century, the trend line returns to a positive slope, as the Romantic composers

from Chopin and Berlioz through Wagner and Brahms introduced ever more complexity in their melodic constructions. For instance, the opening theme to the first movement of Liszt's *Faust Symphony* begins G-G#-A-A#-B-C, containing transitions that mostly occur less than 1 percent of the time in the total sample of 15,618 themes. This ascent eventually surpasses that seen earlier when it attains a new peak around 1917—about the time that Arnold Schoenberg and his Vienna school were evolving atonal and serial tone sequences. But thereafter the trend line moved away toward more diatonic compositions, as composers like Prokofiev, Copeland, and Shostakovich backed off from the more daring music of their formative years. Even Schoenberg retreated from the extreme represented by his 1912 *Pierrot Lunaire*, such as his rather more accessible Piano Concerto of 1942. Unfortunately, since the themes sampled were composed no more recently than the middle of this century, we cannot specify the aftermath of this downward thrust, and the simultaneous existence today of both minimalist music and the electronic avant-garde makes qualitative speculation hazardous. Nonetheless, it is worth pointing out that the observed historical trend complies quite nicely with what musicologists have long held to be the transhistorical changes in melodic chromaticism (e.g., Apel, 1969). Clearly, originality must increase in proportion to chromaticism, for chromatic notes tend to comprise rare two-note transitions, the only real exception to this rule being the F#-G transition, a favorite route by which composers slide into the dominant.

6. Not only does the expected level of melodic originality change over the course of music history, but in addition this characteristic tends to shift in a sensible fashion within works composed in the larger forms. Trend analyses in fact reveal that melodic originality in multiple-movement works tends to be a curvilinear, backward-J function of the order of the movement in which the theme appears (Simonton, 1987b). In concrete terms, the first movement features the most striking themes, the last movement the second most original, whereas the least remarkable melodies are located in the middle one or two movements, on the average. This empirical tendency, of course, follows closely the structure usually seen in the larger instrumental forms, symphonies, quartets, trios, and sonatas, especially. A dramatic and rousing opening movement, commonly in sonata-allegro form, is often succeeded by one or two middle movements in *aba*

song form (including the minuet and trio or scherzo in four-movement works), and then the composition is given the capstone of an exciting finale, most frequently in sonata-allegro or rondo form. The within-composition trend in melodic originality merely provides the gist of this more complex shift in formal structure.

    7. Melodic originality enables us to predict why some compositions are praised as masterpieces whereas others, even when created by the same composer, are condemned as mere occasion pieces. First, computer-generated scores on melodic originality correspond with how compositions are evaluated by musicologists. For instance, Halsey (1976) assessed some 4101 compositions on two five-point scales, one gauging "aesthetic significance" and the other "listener accessibility." The content analytical measure correlates positively with the first of these assessments and negatively with the second (Simonton, 1986, 1989). In other words, the more unpredictable the melodic structure of the themes comprising a work, the higher the piece scores subjectively in profundity and meaningfulness but the lower it scores in easy listening. Second, for those who distrust experts, we can look at the actual repertoire and ask whether melodic originality corresponds in any manner with how frequently a work is performed and recorded. Therefore, an objective measure of "repertoire popularity" was devised by consulting music anthologies, recording catalogues, program guides, music appreciation texts, and a host of kindred sources (Simonton, 1980b), obtaining an index that corresponded with how often a work is really heard by aficionados of classical music (Simonton, 1983a). Interestingly, although repertoire popularity correlates positively with aesthetic significance, it also correlates positively with listener accessibility (Simonton, 1989), indicating that a true masterwork is one of those rare compositions that manages somehow to combine the best of both worlds, importance with approachability. In any event, a composition's popularity was found to be a curvilinear (inverted backward-J) function of melodic originality (Simonton, 1980b). The most successful pieces are those that contain themes in the middle range of melodic originality, lines spiced with just a few quirky jumps and chromaticisms. The trite and mundane melodies that hug the diatonic scale are far too predictable to inspire durable interest, whereas the wildly ambiguous melodic structures of highly chromatic, even atonal themes prove far too intimidating to invite a broad appreciation. However, if the contest is between the overly simple and

the fearsomely complex, simplicity emerges the victor, resulting in a J-shaped rather than inverted-U function.

8. One final consideration must be added to the preceding conclusion: Rather than estimate a melody's originality with respect to the entire body of classical compositions—what we can style "repertoire melodic originality"—we can alternatively calculate its *zeitgeist* originality by comparing a piece with other works composed at the same time (Simonton, 1980b). If we examine how repertoire popularity varies as a function of this contextually defined measure, we get a U-shaped curve, that is, those themes are most appreciated which seem to violate our expectations regarding the baseline melodic structure in a given stylistic period (Simonton, 1980b). This offers us one response to the eternal question of the relative impact of genius and *zeitgeist* in creative achievements: The most acclaimed works are those which depart from, rather than conform to, the norms of the day. Once when one of Beethoven's Rasoumovsky Quartets was being rehearsed for the first time, a violinist griped about whether this stuff could really be called music. Beethoven responded that "Oh, they are not for you, but for a later age!" (Knight, 1973, p. 67). The Master's retort now seems more prophetic than arrogant!

I hope the foregoing points suffice to convince the skeptic that the computer is capable of capturing a critical feature of musical compositions. The content analytical assessment of melodic originality behaves as we would expect it to for the scores assigned to be taken as indicative of a bona fide property of musical aesthetics. Assuming this validation has been successful, we can now inquire how melodic originality varies according to circumstances in a composer's life, with frequent reference to how Mozart complies with the statistical patterns. Below I inspect the consequences of three crucial realities of life, conditions that impinge on musical geniuses as much as everybody else—stress, aging, and death.

STRESS

It is commonplace in the arts to try to connect the idiosyncrasies of a particular composition with concurrent events in a creator's life. This practice is a favorite of psychobiographers and critics alike. Yet the standard modus operandi is to make these linkages in a qualitative and highly speculative fashion, and even then to do so on a single case. In contrast, a series of empirical investigations have shown how melodic originality is associated with stressful conditions in the lives of many composers, thereby providing a more nomothetic set of conclusions (Simonton, 1980a, 1986, 1987b). These stressors can be grouped into a pair of categories, the impersonal and the personal.

By "impersonal" I mean merely that some stressors are by no means unique to a particular composer but rather affect all composers of a particular time and place indiscriminately. The most conspicuous example is warfare. Composers must often try to work while artillery shells explode around them—as Beethoven experienced during Napoleon's occupation of Vienna—and this is not without consequence for their creative work. The most striking effect is that the melodic originality found in their larger compositions tends to become far more variable, the range increasing between their most predictable and most offbeat themes (Simonton, 1986, 1987b). As a further validation of this discovery, Cerulo (1984) found a somewhat similar effect for composers active in war zones during the Second World War, only using more subjective content analyses. So composers cannot escape the march of history when conceiving their masterpieces: The uncertainty in the larger world is mirrored in the greater variability in their use of melodic originality.

But it is the more "personal" stresses faced by the artist that most attracts our curiosity when trying to come to grips with a composition. For one thing, evidence that melodic originality may increase in those compositions that emerge when the creator is suffering a major physical illness—at least this connection held in the life of Ludwig van Beethoven (Simonton, 1987b). This finding can be best interpreted in conjunction with a second, this one demonstrated on ten top composers, including Mozart: Those periods in which a composer experiences the most stressful events—as determined by a biographical adaptation of a life-change scale (Holmes and Rahe, 1967)—also are prone to be those periods in which melodies become decidedly original (Simonton, 1980a). Hence, both physical and mental distress seem to inspire the production of unpredictable melodic lines. This positive association may be understood as an illustration of the common belief that music, like many other art forms, is a means of emotional communication from creators to appreciators. Because music sounds the way emotions feel, melodies provide a shared metaphor for otherwise private feelings. Consistent with this interpretation is the fact that minor-key melodies, which are popularly taken to convey melancholic moods or tragic emotions—as in Mozart's second G Minor Symphony—score higher in melodic originality than do themes in major keys (Simonton, 1987b). This explanation is also in accord with the emotional tone often attributed to the "blue note" of classic jazz, for this minor third occurs relatively infrequently in the dominant music tradition at the time when the blues first emerged in America.

I realize full well how often it is claimed that Mozart's creativity seemed wonderfully isolated from the trials and tribulations of life. But regarding how melodic originality fluctuated in his thematic material, he follows the same regularity as other musical geniuses (Simonton, 1980a). The one qualification is that he is one of the lucky few whose adolescence and adulthood were not marred by major wars, and thus his stylistic adjustments were insulated from such impersonal stressors.

AGING

As composers advance along their respective careers, the melodic originality that defines the building blocks of their compositions tends to progressively expand (Simonton, 1980b). This upward thrust in personal stylistic development occurs independently of the broader trends in the Western music tradition mentioned earlier, and thus it fits in well with those theories of artistic motivation that assume creators are compelled by the incessant need to generate ever more original works, excelling what has been already accomplished by themselves and others (Martindale, 1990). A peculiar twist occurs in this lifespan developmental transition, however, namely that a modest dip often appears in the progression sometime after a composer's fifty-sixth year of life, as if the constant push toward novelty is weakening (Simonton, 1980b). Since Mozart died twenty years before this anticipated turnaround, we can surmise that the upward quest for melodic originality never ceased during the course of *his* career (Simonton, 1980a).

Another developmental transformation is perhaps even more fascinating. As we have already seen, once we have estimated the general trend of melodic originality from 1500 to 1950, we can easily determine whether any given melody is typical of the musical *zeitgeist* for the year of its creation, arriving at a gauge of a theme's *zeitgeist* originality. This attribute has a provocative relationship with a composer's age, permitting us to link temporal changes in the creator's career with those taking place in the larger world of musical activity: As a composer matures, the *zeitgeist* originality of his or her thematic material progressively grows in a linear manner (Simonton, 1980b). This tendency is most intriguing in light of the debate between genius and *zeitgeist* interpretations of historial change (Simonton, 1984b), for apparently it is only in the early phases of a career that geniuses are dependent upon the *zeitgeist* to dictate their style. As composers proceed along the process of aesthetic self-discovery, they increasingly find their own unique voice, diminishing their intimacy with the musical milieu. Thus a creative career seems to begin with mere imitation of predominant models and to end in complete self-actualization. Mozart's symphonic output may be taken as typical of this developmental trend. His works start as precocious and competent but entirely tame reflections of the musical vogue, yet eventually in his last three symphonies, the thirty-ninth through forty-first, he produced compositions boasting no audience amongst his contemporaries, and looking more toward the future than the present.

DEATH

Historiometric studies of historical figures have often detected curious transformations that take place in the concluding years of life. For one thing, such individuals undergo a simplification of their thought processes, as if the goal was to unclutter the mind in the final days (Suedfeld and Piedrahita, 1984). This shift occurs only if the individuals in question can foresee the approach of death, owing to severe deterioration of their physical health, such as a terminal illness. Another change is that creators will frequently exhibit a resurgence of output as they near their final days, suggesting that they complete all the projects that have been circulating within their heads before it becomes impossible to do so (Simonton, 1990a). In the specific domain of classical music, such developmental deviations may be part of a larger complex of changes known as the *swan-song phenomenon* (Simonton, 1989). According to an analysis of 1919 compositions by 172 classical composers, right before a composer's death, melodic originality declines very rapidly, a "terminal drop" that is quite independent of the creator's actual chronological age. Furthermore, this downturn is part of an array of reversals that distinguish a composer's last works. For example, the compositions that are conceived in the final years tend to be, on the average, shorter while still scoring higher in aesthetic significance and becoming more frequently performed in the classical repertoire. In a nutshell, when a composer must face the frightening truth of death, the odds increase that they will produce brief, simple, and yet profound pieces that serve as popular capstones of their creative careers. Perhaps having undergone a life review, they endeavor to create a final artistic testament that helps secure their place with posterity.

The swan-song phenomenon is a function not of a composer's actual age, but solely of the number of years remaining before death. Therefore, so long as a composer can have a premonition of life's end, last-works' effects will be evident. Thus Schubert, who was severely afflicted with syphilis, could produce swan songs (including the songs collected posthumously to form the cycle entitled *Schwanengesang*), just as Tchaikovsky, anticipating the necessity of taking his own life, could compose a suicide note (the Sixth Symphony). In contrast, Chausson, who rammed his head into a wall after losing control of his bicycle, would not be expected to display such a stylistic switch. It follows that Mozart, though only in his mid-thirties, could be expected to create swan songs once he began to contemplate death on the horizon. While several works in his final year might be suggested as possibilities—most notably the *Ave Verum Corpus* of June 17—the most obvious choice is the *Requiem* which, because of the mysterious circumstances of its commissioning, Mozart thought might be his own. As is well known, he only finished the first 12 of the 15 sections before dying, and it was the sole piece he was working on in the final days, frequently in a desperate race against fate. Actually, I would point to one section of the *Requiem* as the core exemplar of what we are seeking: the chorus "Lacrymosa," a setting of the Latin text describing the tears shed as one prepares to leave this life and face God's judgment. To set these poignant words Mozart conjured up a "melody almost too limpid for choral singing" (Blom, 1974, p. 181). On the afternoon of December 4, 1791, the day before Mozart passed away, he gathered some friends to sing through the *Requiem*, he himself taking the alto part. But when the chorus reached the opening lines of the "Lacrymosa," he could not help breaking down, and laid the score aside to weep. Not too much later paralysis set in, and less than an hour after the midnight of the next day, Mozart was dead. How might this scene have better served Milos Forman's movie *Amadeus*!

MOZART AS PROTOTYPICAL GENIUS

Let me reiterate that when we compare Mozart against the profile of musical genius, we should never expect him to match our nomothetic expectations perfectly. There will always be exceptions to every rule, just as in English orthography the principle "*i* before *e* except after *c*, or when sounded like *a* as in *neighbor* and *weigh*" will run afoul on many *weird* words. Nevertheless, I think it should be clear by now that according to numerous criteria Mozart represents the prototype of musical genius. His own life and work dovetails so closely with the lives and works of the entire set of classical masters that it is hard to resist the temptation to make him the touchstone against which all other composers, even those of the caliber of Beethoven or Bach, may be judged. Indeed, I would like to argue that if it were not for one single exception, Mozart would have no rivals for the uppermost spot on anyone's list of musical giants. That exception is his abnormally early demise. Although he may have earned a few credits with posterity for such a premature end—due to a well-documented tragic-death effect (Simonton, 1976, 1984b, 1990b)—the net repercussion of this happenstance is most likely negative. Why?

Historiometric studies show that achievers who begin their creative activities at exceptionally youthful ages are also prone to produce much later in life, and to be more prolific the entire length of their careers (Simonton, 1988a), a set of intercorrelations that hold just as well in the specific case of classical music (Simonton, 1990b). On this basis alone, we must predict that, had Mozart lived until the early 1820s, many more masterpieces would have come from his hand, in all likelihood more total works than credited to the assiduous J. S. Bach. These additions to the Köchel catalog would have necessarily augmented Mozart's already intimidating reputation. To put this point in perspective, where would Beethoven be without the over two decades extra life span he had over Mozart? Can we even imagine a Beethoven without the Fifth through Ninth symphonies, the Emperor Concerto, the Archduke Trio, *An die ferne Geliebte*, the *Missa Solemnis*, or, to my mind especially, the late-period string quartets and piano sonatas? And where would Bach stand in the charts without *The Well-Tempered Clavier*, and the *Goldberg Variations*, the *Brandenburg Concerti*, the *St. Matthew Passion*, the Christmas and Easter oratorios, *A Musical Offering*, and *The Art of the Fugue*?

I believe it is a truism to state that Mozart promised to be the greatest musical genius of all time. What makes me even more confident of this affirmation are two other items discerned from the empirical studies. First, because he died about five years short of the usual career optimum, it was very probable that his best compositions still lay before him at the time he passed away; his most popular opera, his most monumental symphony, his most profound quintet, quartet, and sonata, and possibly his most moving *Requiem* remain forever in some limbo of merely hypothetical existence (even if we allow that computers may some day be programmed to simulate his genius). Second, if Mozart followed the pattern of musical geniuses generally, he would have separated himself ever further from the musical *zeitgeist* of his day, his distinctive musical personality evolving in unpredictable directions. After more fully assimilating all forms and techniques, and perhaps allowing himself to be enlarged by the middle-period Beethoven, there would eventually emerge a late-period Mozart, his melancholy rendered deeper and more wise. It is quite possible, therefore, to conceive that Mozart, and not Beethoven, would have become the composer responsible for revolutionizing music. Mozart rather than Beethoven would have been the first composer to strike out on an aesthetic mission free of the dictates of patrons. It would have been Mozart, not Beethoven, who straddled the two worlds of classical and romantic styles, providing the unparalleled transition figure who initiates one tradition by culminating another.

And where would Weber's contribution reside if Mozart had the opportunity to develop German opera beyond *The Magic Flute*? Where would Schubert's reputation dwell had Mozart cast his songs in a more advanced Mozartian style? And what would Rossini have done if that predecessor he so much admired had been able to follow up *The Marriage of Figaro* with his very own *Barber of Seville*? Had Mozart lived only as long as the average composer, he would have been still standing like a colossus while Beethoven, Weber, Schubert, Rossini, and many other notables of the early nineteenth century struggled to establish their personal styles. If even Haydn, over twenty years Mozart's senior, could not help but be affected by Mozart's genius, surely the impression Mozart would have made on the musical development of the early Romantics would have been equally profound. Under such circumstances, who dares doubt that Mozart would have been universally proclaimed, in his own day and ours, as the musical genius *sui generis*?

REFERENCES

Albert, R. S. (1975), Toward a behavioral definition of genius. *Amer. Psychologist*, 30:140–151.

—— (1980), Family positions and the attainment of eminence: A study of special family positions and special family experiences. *Gifted Child Quart.*, 24:87–95.

Apel, W. (1969), *Harvard Dictionary of Music*, 2nd ed. Cambridge, MA: Harvard University Press.

Barlow, H., & Morgenstern, S. (1948), *A Dictionary of Musical Themes*. New York: Crown.

—— (1976), *A Dictionary of Opera and Song Themes*, rev. ed. New York: Crown.

Berlyne, D. E. (1971), *Aesthetics and Psychobiology*. New York: Appleton-Century-Crofts.

Bliss, W. D. (1970), Birth order of creative writers. *J. Individ. 'Psychol.*, 26:200–202.

Blom, E. (1974), *Mozart*. London: Dent.

Cerulo, K. A. (1984), Social disruption and its effects on music: An empirical analysis. *Soc. Forces*, 62:885–904.

Cox, C. (1926), *The Early Mental Traits of Three Hundred Geniuses*. Stanford, CA: Stanford University Press.

Dennis, W. (1955), Variations in productivity among creative workers. *Scient. Monthly*, 80:277–278.

Eisenstadt, J. M. (1978), Parental loss and genius. *Amer. Psychologist*, 33:211–223.

Ellis, H. (1904), *A Study of British Genius*. London: Hurst & Blackett.

Farnsworth, P. R. (1969), *The Social Psychology of Music*, 2nd ed. Ames: Iowa State University Press.

Feldman, D. (1986), *Nature's Gambit*. New York: Basic Books.

Galton, F. (1869), *Hereditary Genius: An Inquiry into Its Causes and Consequences*. London: Macmillan.

—— (1874), *English Men of Science: Their Nature and Nurture*. London: Macmillan.

Halsey, R. S. (1976), *Classical Music Recordings for Home and Library*. Chicago: American Library Association.

Hayes, J. R. (1989), *The Complete Problem Solver*, 2nd ed. Hillsdale, NJ: Lawrence Erlbaum.

Hollingworth, L. (1926), *Gifted Children*. New York: Macmillan.

Holmes, T. S., & Rahe, R. H. (1967), The social adjustment rating scale. *J. Psychosom. Res.*, 11:213–218.

Knight, F. (1973), *Beethoven and the Age of Revolution*. New York: International Publishers.

Martindale, C. (1990), *The Clockwork Muse: The Predictability of Artistic Change*. New York: Basic Books.

——— Uemura, A. (1983), Stylistic evolution in European music. *Leonardo*, 16:225–228.

McClelland, D. C. (1973), Testing for competence rather than for "intelligence." *Amer. Psychologist*, 28:1–14.

Moles, A. (1958), *Information Theory and Esthetic Perception*, trans. J. E. Cohen. Urbana: University of Illinois Press, 1968.

Murray, P., ed. (1989), *Genius: The History of an Idea*. Oxford, U.K.: Blackwell.

Paisley, W. J. (1964), Identifying the unknown communicator in painting, literature and music: The significance of minor encoding habits. *J. Comm.*, 14:219–237.

Schubert, D. S. P., Wagner, M. E., & Schubert, H. J. P. (1977), Family constellation and creativity: Firstborn predominance among classical music composers. *J. Psychol.*, 95:147–149.

Simonton, D. K. (1975), Sociocultural context of individual creativity: A transhistorical time-series analysis. *J. Person. Social Psychol.*, 32:1119–1133.

——— (1976), Biographical determinants of achieved eminence: A multivariate approach to the Cox data. *J. Person. Social Psychol.*, 33:218–226.

——— (1977a), Creative productivity, age, and stress: A biographical time-series analysis of 10 classical composers. *J. Person. Social Psychol.*, 35:791–804.

——— (1977b), Eminence, creativity, and geographic marginality: A recursive structural equation model. *J. Person. Social Psychol.*, 35:805–816.

——— (1980a), Thematic fame and melodic originality in classical music: A multivariate computer-content analysis. *J. Person.*, 48:206–219.

——— (1980b), Thematic fame, melodic originality, and musical zeitgeist: A biographical and transhistorical content analysis. *J. Person. Social Psychol.*, 38:972–983.

——— (1983a), Esthetics, biography, and history in musical creativity. In: *Documentary Report on the Ann Arbor Symposium on the Application of Psychology to the Teaching and Learning of Music: Session III. Motivation and Creativity*. Reston, VA: Music Educators National Conference, pp. 41–48.

——— (1983b), Intergenerational transfer of individual differences in hereditary monarchs: Genes, role-modeling, cohort, or sociocultural effects? *J. Person. Social Psychol.*, 44:354–364.

——— (1984a), Artistic creativity and interpersonal relationships across and within generations. *J. Person. Social Psychol.*, 46:1273–1286.

——— (1984b), *Genius, Creativity, and Leadership: Historiometric Inquiries*. Cambridge, MA: Harvard University Press.

——— (1984c), Melodic structure and note transition probabilities: A content analysis of 15,618 classical themes. *Psychol. Music*, 12:3–16.

—— (1986), Aesthetic success in classical music: A computer analysis of 1935 compositions. *Emp. Stud. Arts*, 4:1–17.

—— (1987a), Developmental antecedents of achieved eminence. *Annals Child Develop.*, 5:131–169.

—— (1987b), Musical aesthetics and creativity in Beethoven: A computer analysis of 105 compositions. *Emp. Stud. Arts*, 5:87–104.

—— (1988a), Age and outstanding achievement: What do we know after a century of research? *Psychol. Bull.*, 104:251–267.

—— (1988b), Galtonian genius, Kroeberian configurations, and emulation: A generational time-series analysis of Chinese civilization. *J. Person. Social Psychol.*, 55:230–238.

—— (1988c), *Scientific Genius: A Psychology of Science.* Cambridge, U.K.: Cambridge University Press.

—— (1989), The swan-song phenomenon: Last-works effects for 172 classical composers. *Psychol. & Aging*, 4:42–47.

—— (1990a), Creativity in the later years: Optimistic prospects for achievement. *Gerontologist*, 30:626–631.

—— (1990b), *Psychology, Science, and History: An Introduction to Historiometry.* New Haven, CT: Yale University Press.

—— (1991a), Career landmarks in science: Individual differences and interdisciplinary contrasts. *Devel. Psychol.*, 27:119–130.

—— (1991b), Emergence and realization of genius: The lives and works of 120 classical composers. *J. Person. Social Psychol.*, 61:829–840.

—— (1991c), Latent-variable models of posthumous reputation: A quest for Galton's *G. J. Person. Social Psychol.*, 60:607–619.

Stewart, L. H. (1977), Birth order and political leadership. In: *The Psychological Examination of Political Leaders*, ed. M. G. Hermann. New York: Free Press, pp. 205–236.

Suedfeld, P., & Piedrahita, L. E. (1984), Intimations of mortality: Integrative Simplification as a predictor of death. *J. Person. Social Psychol.*, 47:848–852.

Terman, L. M. (1917), The intelligence quotient of Francis Galton in childhood. *Amer. J. Psychol.*, 28:209–215.

—— (1925), *Mental and Physical Traits of a Thousand Gifted Children.* Stanford, CA: Stanford University Press.

—— Oden, M. H. (1959), *The Gifted Group at Mid-Life.* Stanford, CA: Stanford University Press.

2

Mozart as Prodigy, Mozart as Artifact

David Henry Feldman, Ph.D.

INTRODUCTION

It hardly needs to be said that Mozart stands almost alone among the most legendary prodigies of Western culture. In almost any discussion of extreme talent and its fulfillment, the name Mozart comes up early and often. In a sense, Mozart defines what it means to be a prodigy: Astounding talent, astonishingly early productivity at the highest levels, and a powerful personality seem to capture the essence of the prodigy (Feldman, 1986). Yet, the idea we in Western culture tend to hold of the prodigy has not always been as it is today. Indeed, the earliest meaning of the word referred to a portent or sign, usually of a cataclysmic change, that was "out of the usual course of nature."

In this essay, we will explore two sets of issues. First we will examine the prodigy Mozart in relation to the small but growing body of knowledge that is accumulating about prodigies in various fields; and second, we will examine the way in which our image of Mozart is conditioned by the images we hold of the prodigy, images that have become part of our culture, thus cultural artifacts although conceptual ones.

[1]*Acknowledgments.* Based on a presentation at the Symposium: "The Pleasures and Perils of Genius: Mostly Mozart" held at the University of California, San Francisco, June 7–9, 1991. I would like to thank Peter Ostwald, M.D., the convener of the meeting, both for inviting me to participate and for his longstanding interest in my work. Support from the Jessie Smith Noyes Foundation, the Exxon Foundation, and the Grant Foundation is also gratefully acknowledged.

MOZART AS PRODIGY

It could be argued that since Mozart is *the* prodigy of history, the way to approach the question of Mozart as prodigy is to compare other prodigies to Mozart to see how well *they* fit the pattern. To the degree that other cases resemble Mozart in mind, body, and spirit, would those cases be appropriately called prodigies? Although arguments could certainly be made for taking this approach, it will not be the one taken here. The main reason for not taking this approach is suggested by the title of the second part of the present discussion; namely, that our knowledge of Mozart is filtered through a set of cultural myths and expectations that may have little to do with the actual person who lived from 1756 to 1791 and who was named Wolfgang Mozart. To use what we now *believe* was true of Mozart as our yardstick prejudges the outcome of our inquiry. We wish, after all, to know better the nature of the prodigy, not to force other cases to conform to what we happen to believe is true of *the* prodigy.

As it happens, the author and his colleagues have been studying actual, living cases of children who have demonstrated early prodigious tendencies, children as young as 3 years of age. This research covered a period of more than a decade and followed six children and their families from childhood through adolescence. Our experiences in studying the prodigies and their families have been reported at length elsewhere (Feldman, 1986); for the purposes of the present discussion, I will distill what we have learned into ten points which seem to be true of prodigies.

Having this list of ten qualities or characteristics of prodigies will permit us to compare what is known about the young Mozart with this empirically derived template. From this effort we will be able to see just how canonical a prodigy Mozart really was, given the limitations on what we can know about him after two hundred years.

Getting Mozart to conform to any kind of preexisting mold could be seen as sacrilege, but it should be emphasized that this is not at all my purpose. Nothing that I might do as an exercise in defining the nature of the prodigy will reduce Mozart's unique place in history. Mozart was Mozart. Still, if we can compare what we know about Mozart with what we know about other extremely talented children, it is possible that we may serve the twin purposes of knowing Mozart just a bit better, on the one hand, and knowing a bit more about prodigies, on the other. Although it is unlikely that there will ever be another Mozart, it is fair to suppose that many promising talents have been lost over the centuries because of a lack of knowledge about how to discover and nurture them (Gardner, 1992).

Now we will turn to the ten characteristics that seem to be emerging from the literature on prodigies, a literature that includes fewer than twenty cases actually studied while they were children (Revesz, 1925; Baumgarten, 1930; Feldman, 1986). In addition, there have been biographical and autobiographical accounts of cases that enrich and enhance the data base (Menuhin, 1977; Ostwald, 1991).

1. FAMILY HISTORY

By and large, when you find a prodigy you also find a family history of interest in the field in which the prodigy appears. The same tends to be true of very high level performers who were not prodigies (Bloom, 1985). If a child performs exceptionally well in a sport, he or she usually comes from a family that has been involved in sports for several generations. Musical prodigies tend to come from families where music is and has been a central passion; the legendary Bach family is perhaps the most striking example.

Mozart was not an exception to this rule, but neither was he from a family of musicians going back several generations. Until the generation before Wolfgang, the family could boast few musicians, none of them prominent; artisans and bricklayers were the predominant trades of Mozart's forebears on both sides. Mozart's grandfather on his mother's side was a musician: "He studied at the Benedictine University of Salzburg, and there acquired not only book learning but also experience with music. His appointment as bass in the choir and instructor of singing at the monastery school of St. Peter's affords evidence of his musical talent" (Schenk, 1955, p. 6). Mozart's maternal grandmother was the daughter of a musician.

On his father's side, there is no evidence of musical talent until Mozart's father Leopold pursued a career as a court musician and church instructor. Leopold's role in Wolfgang's life has of course been the subject of great attention and not a small amount of speculation, but what is of note in the context of the point under consideration is that his father was the first musician in his family, an unusually recent appearance of strong musical talent where prodigies are concerned.

Thus, although there is clear evidence that interest in music of more than a passing sort existed on both sides of the Mozart family, that interest appeared relatively close to Wolfgang's generation: two generations earlier on his mother's side, while only a generation earlier on his father's side. For most prodigies the line runs longer, wider, and deeper in the specific field or a closely related one.

2. SPECIFIC TALENTS

Although prodigies are exceptionally talented, these talents tend to be relatively focused within a specific area. Prodigies are not generalists who could do well in any field; they are rather more specialists who happen to be blessed with a specific gift that permits them to accomplish great heights within a relatively constrained domain. In my study of six male prodigies, their IQs were estimated to range from a low of 115 or 120 to a high of over 200. Reports about other cases are consistent with my data; prodigies are not necessarily possessed of extremely high IQs, although they tend to be bright.

If the prodigy's specific gift for music or art or mathematics or chess were not supported by at least a reasonable degree of general alertness, we would in all likelihood be dealing with a *savant* rather than a prodigy. A savant is someone whose functioning is very low in general, but who exhibits incredible facility in a specific realm. Music is one kind of ability found in savants, but they may also show remarkable memory capacity, drawing skill, calculation or calendar skills that border on the uncanny (Howe, 1989; Treffert, 1989). There are those who have characterized Mozart as little more than a savant; certainly that is the impression one gets in, for example, Peter Shaffer's (1982) play *Amadeus* and the Milos Forman (1984) film based on that play as well. We will come back to this point in the second part of the discussion, where the image of Mozart as a savant can be seen as an overly zealous corrective to the equally distorted image of him as perfection itself.

In Mozart's case, it seems clear that he was reasonably bright in certain areas other than music; reasonably bright but certainly not exceptional. We know that he picked up a good speaking and reading knowledge of several languages other than his native German, and we know that as a boy he was passionate about mathematics for a time; but we also know that his intellectual life was neither deep in the conventional sense, nor wide. His interests were dominated by music, and his talents, while extending beyond music, were overshadowed and controlled by musical purposes.

A contemporary of Mozart's who traveled in the same social circles, Karoline Pichler, wrote about him (and also Haydn) as "persons who displayed in their contacts with others absolutely no other extraordinary intellectual capacity and almost no kind of intellectual training, of scientific or higher education. . . . Silly jokes, and in the case of Mozart an irresponsible way of life, were all that they displayed to their fellow men" (Pichler, 1844, cited by Landon, 1990, p. 107).

The majesty of the mature Mozart's musical gifts cannot be disputed. There is also ample evidence of the power of the talents that were developed during his first two decades. Mozart's fingers, for example, were exceptionally strong, and his command over musical form so complete that other musicians marveled at it. But these gifts were highly specific to music, and Mozart, like so many other prodigies, probably could not have distinguished himself in anything other than music.

3. FIRST-BORN MALES

The prodigy tradition has been a male tradition, particularly a first-born male tradition (Goldsmith, 1987). In some groups, such as the Hasidic Jews, the focus of resources on first-born males is an explicit part of the culture. In other groups the bias toward oldest sons is not explicit, but holds true nonetheless; an example would be in European culture where laws of inheritance and privilege single out oldest sons for preferential treatment. Not surprisingly, prodigies tended to be first-born sons as well (Rolfe, 1978).

There is of course the question of the extent to which these traditions of exclusion of girls and later-born boys are based on biological versus cultural realities, a question which cannot be fully answered. What is true is that there has never been a culture where truly unbiased conditions exist, making it impossible to find out to what extent biological talents differ in kind and strength among children in various places in the order of birth and of differing genders (Goldsmith, 1987). It must be added as well that the fields in which prodigies have appeared have tended to be male-dominated ones such as chess, mathematics, and music, although these fields are changing rapidly.

Mozart was not a first-born son. He was the second of two surviving children (among seven births), five years younger than his sister Nannerl. His older sister benefited from the presence of a music teacher father, and was taught from about age 7 to play the clavier and to read music. It was Nannerl's involvement in music, in fact, that provided the "crystallizing experience" for 3-year-old Wolfgang (Feldman, 1971, 1974; Walters and Gardner, 1986). Wolfgang was present as Nannerl practiced her music, and he quickly became fascinated. His amazing musical talent was obvious to his father and to other musicians who visited the Mozart home before Wolfgang was 4 years old.

Therefore, in Mozart's case, having an older sister actually served to facilitate his musical development rather than drain resources away from it. As it happened, Nannerl was very talented and very generous, helping her younger brother and fostering his interest in music. But she was not as talented as Wolfgang, nor did she have the passion for music that he did. Before long Nannerl's role became that of support and companionship. Rather than competition for resources, she added to the richness of Mozart's musical world. This exception indeed proves the rule about first-born sons; that is, the focus of the process was on the little boy, and his sister contributed to that process.

It is interesting (but perhaps futile) to speculate on what might have happened to Mozart if his older sibling had been a boy, particularly a boy with ambitious goals and a competitive spirit. The effect would probably have been to reduce the likelihood that Wolfgang would have done the great work that we commemorated in 1991, two hundred years after his death. It is possible that he would have composed *The Magic Flute* or *Don Giovanni* anyway, but it would have been less likely.

Thus, in Mozart's case, he violates a general rule about prodigies, but in doing so, actually tends to strengthen the generalization that prodigies are usually first-born males. Perhaps it would be more accurate to restate the rule to say that prodigies appear in families where there is a focus of resources on the most promising talent, which, historically, was assumed to be located in first-born sons.

4. SUFFICIENT RESOURCES

There are many other potential prodigies than there are actual prodigies. The main reason for the relatively small number of actual prodigies, other than the rarity of extreme talent itself, is the unavailability of sufficient resources to sustain the process of talent development or the unwillingness to use those resources for such purposes (Hayes, 1981).

It is probably a safe assumption that the pool of talent extends across virtually all ethnic groups, classes, and cultures. Yet the vast majority of prodigies come from relatively well off families, from the middle and upper classes, and from certain cultures. Of my six subjects, five were from comfortably well off families, while one family lived well but on minimal resources. Mozart's family, while not wealthy, was comfortably middle class. Mozart's father made a good living as a music teacher, was ambitious, and was willing to commit the family's resources to the development of Wolfgang's talent.

Few realize that the process of bringing a promising talent to full power is one that takes at least ten years (Hayes, 1981; Gardner, 1991). Even the most extreme cases, and Mozart was certainly one of these, require substantial resources for at least a decade. While many families are willing to make a commitment to support a child's talent for a year or two, it takes an unusual set of parents (in practice, one parent tends to be directly involved while the other serves a support role) to stay the course long enough to find out if a child's promise will be fulfilled in adolescence and adulthood. One of my own cases, a very gifted young chess player, abandoned the game when his father lost his sense of resolve and became less willing to transport his son to chess matches (Feldman, 1986).

Mozart never went to school. His father devoted virtually all of his time and money to preparing the young Wolfgang for what he hoped would be a lucrative career as a court musician. Although Leopold's vision was limited (he never realized how transcendent his son's gift for composition was), and although he was motivated as much by the goal of moving into the nobility and the monied classes as he was by a love of music, Leopold provided an extraordinary musical education for Wolfgang.

Other interests and subjects such as languages and mathematics were not ignored, but were learned in the context of whatever served

Mozart's musical career. Thus Mozart received the kind of education he needed to develop the full power of his talent, and he received it for as long as was required. In fact, the eventual tension between father and son was substantially over whether or not Wolfgang had received sufficient training and experience to go off on his own (Hildesheimer, 1977). At age 17 Wolfgang felt ready to take his place among working musicians. His father, knowing better than Wolfgang the treacherous path ahead, tried to maintain control over his son's activities for several more years (Schenk, 1955).

In the area of resources then, Mozart conforms well to the image that has emerged of the prodigy as the focal point in a support system. Often schooled outside formal institutions, often the recipient of the vast proportion of a family's resources (both material and psychic), often protected and directed toward a career from an early age, and often seen as a future source of wealth and fame for the family, the prodigy becomes the sun in a small solar system, except that the prodigy *receives* energy from all the other bodies in the system rather than sustaining them (Menuhin, 1977; Rolfe, 1978). Wolfgang Mozart was no exception to this rule.

5. SINGLE-MINDEDNESS

In the cases I have studied, one of the most striking qualities found among the six boys was a powerful desire toward becoming the best in whatever field they were pursuing, which ranged from writing to chess to science to music. The quality was a mixture of passion for the knowledge and challenge their chosen domain presented, along with a kind of ambitiousness that would brook little compromise (Feldman, 1986). They also seemed to have an internal barometer or gyroscope that would let them know when they were on course and when they had veered from it.

Compared with my own subjects, and with the cases I have read in the literature, Mozart was single-minded but not in quite the same way as most other prodigies. It is without doubt true that his passion for music was pervasive; his whole life was organized around music. It is said that Mozart continued to compose his D-Minor Quartet in 1783 as his wife Constanze gave birth in the next room (Schenk, 1955). The story cannot be verified, but the quality of single-mindedness it bespeaks comes through in many sources. There is little doubt that when it came to composing, Mozart could not be distracted from his task. Although he did not always meet his deadlines, he seemed to be following an internal agenda that governed much of his life as a composer.

Yet, it is also true that Mozart was probably the most social and gregarious prodigy of all time. To a number of observers, Mozart's social life was so varied and so full that his record of productivity is hard to believe. Malcolm Boyd wrote in *The Mozart Compendium* (1990) that: "Mozart enjoyed a wide circle of friends, acquaintances, relatives, colleagues and pupils—so wide, indeed, that one sometimes wonders how he found time to compose" (cited by Landon, 1990, p. 41). His circle included hundreds of people with whom he had frequent contact; he enjoyed billiards, darts, shooting, walking in the park, riding his horse, and various games of chance. He attended innumerable social events, many of which were professional obligations but many of which were not.

As I have discussed at greater length elsewhere (Feldman, 1992), Mozart stands apart from virtually every other known prodigy in being the most social, although it must also be added that his relationships with other people were in many ways peculiar. One possible way to reconcile his musical preoccupations with his seeming sociability was offered by Hildesheimer, who observed that: "Mozart's reticence about personalities is so striking that it inclines us to think he saw in his fellow man only what was relevant to him, the musical side of the personality" (1983, p. 26). Hildesheimer (1977) also wrote that: "He [Mozart] himself never had sufficient sensitivity to assess how people responded to him. Approachability and inaccessibility were qualities that Mozart did not register in his relationships; in the realm of human contact, he was always a helpless foreigner" (p. 95).

Therefore, while it can be said with confidence that Mozart was as driven toward musical greatness as any prodigy, it must also be said that the form that drive took was unique. To the casual observer it may often have seemed that Mozart was frivolous and lazy, inclined more toward partying than working. There is of course a surface truth to this observation, but it seems too facile to describe Mozart as lacking in discipline. It would be hard to account for his hundreds of compositions if he were anything other than single-minded, albeit in a way that is rarely seen among prodigies (Davies, 1989).

6. INNER CONFIDENCE

Related to single-mindedness, a quality that I saw in my own subjects had to do with a sense of the power of their gift; I labeled it inner confidence (Feldman, 1986). As early as 3 or 4, my subjects seemed to sense that they were carrying a special ability to do something. When they encountered the field that allowed this internal ability to express itself, a rapid engagement and passionate embracing of that field usually followed. The quality is often mistakenly seen as arrogance, but in my experience it is less arrogance than confidence based on something real and genuine.

For Mozart, that he possessed a quality something like inner confidence seems very likely. His understanding of his own abilities was amazing, and his views of other musicians were uncanny in their accuracy. As early as 7 or 8 he was describing various musicians with sometimes devastating accuracy. Emily Anderson's (1966) edition of Mozart's letters contains numerous examples of Wolfgang's confident sense of himself in relation to those with whom he came into contact through music. It is well known that he truly admired only a tiny number of fellow musicians: Haydn, Bach, and few others.

Mozart never seemed to doubt his ability to perform and compose at the very highest levels (Jahn, 1891; Gardner, 1992). If he had even fleeting doubts, they are not to be found in his letters (Lang, 1963). He certainly experienced disappointment, even despair at times, but never were his more difficult moments caused by doubts about the gifts he knew he possessed. It cannot be proven, of course, that Mozart's confidence was never shaken, but this quality is consistent with what has been found in several other cases, giving support to the belief that Mozart too experienced a kind of inner confidence that helped sustain him during his many difficult periods.

7. A "MIDLIFE CRISIS" DURING ADOLESCENCE

As observed by Jeanne Bamberger (1982, 1992), a student of musical development, most prodigies experience a crisis in their lives sometime during adolescence. This crisis seems to be a function of changes both internal, having to do with their understanding of their own mental processes, and external, having to do with the realization that they must soon make their way as adults.

The one case in my own study who pursued a career in classical music during the period I observed him, may have been a rare exception to Bamberger's rule (Feldman, 1986). Although he did go through a difficult transition between his tenth and twelfth years, switching from composer to performer, his adolescence was not marked by the kind of crisis that Bamberger so vividly describes. This was the case also with Mozart, although perhaps for different reasons. Mozart does not seem to have confronted his own mental processes at all, or at least there is little evidence that he did.

From the evidence that is available, primarily his letters, Mozart does not appear to have been a reflective person. His life was of course lived in an era before psychology and psychoanalysis were part of cultural life, but many of his contemporaries were philosophically inclined; apparently, Wolfgang was not. Although he lived during a period when the ideas that gave rise to the Enlightenment were hotly discussed, and during which many major world events took place (e.g., the French Revolution), Mozart's world revolved around musical matters.

There was a late adolescent crisis in Mozart's life, but it did not involve a questioning of his musical abilities, nor did it involve confronting the adult world of professional musicians. Mozart fell hopelessly in love with a young singer named Aloysia Weber and wanted to pursue his relationship with her instead of pursuing his own musical career (Nohl, 1893). In a series of letters between Wolfgang and his father, it is clear that Wolfgang tried to break free of his father's influence (at the same time as he needed his father's help). This period was probably the beginning of what became a strained relationship right up until Mozart's father died in 1787.

The midlife crisis, so called because it occurs in most prodigies after ten or more years of intense pursuit of mastery in their chosen domain, appears not to have occurred in Mozart, although, as noted, another crisis did occur. Interestingly, this crisis was more in the interpersonal sphere than in relation to his sense of his own competence as a musician. Consistent with Mozart's involvements in the world of other people, in some ways it seems to fit what we know of him that he would face a late adolescent crisis because of how he felt about another person, not how he felt about his music.

8. Ten or More Years to Develop Talent

A frequent belief about prodigies is that their talent comes fully formed, requiring little or no instruction for its expression. While it cannot be denied that there are powerful biological underpinnings to the extreme talents found in all prodigies, it is now absolutely clear that, contrary to myth, a prodigy requires vast amounts of effort from those who would guide his or her development. In particular, the role of mentors and teachers is utterly central; without sustained, coordinated, and caring attention, a prodigy's potential will almost certainly not reach full expression.

From the work of John Hayes (1981), among others, we know that it takes at least ten years for a novice to achieve mastery over any domain. Even in the most extreme cases, this rule seems to hold true. Another observer of extreme development in prodigies and others, Howard Gardner, has written about this surprisingly constant ten-year period of development: "The facts of career development are quite striking. Independent of domain, it takes about ten years of intensive training for the young individual to master the tools of his or her trade, to belong to the cohort of well trained practitioners of a calling . . ." (Gardner, 1991, p. 5). Mozart was about 3 when he started his musical training; this was an unusually young age, but it still took more than ten years even for Mozart to reach for the stars in his compositions.

The first known compositions of Mozart are little minuets, written down by his father Leopold in his sister Nannerl's composition book, from his fourth, fifth, and sixth years. Although extraordinary, the compositions between his sixth and sixteenth years have not stood the test of time in the sense that, were they not those of Mozart, we would be unlikely to know about them. They are in this sense of historical interest only, or of interest as sources of information about Mozart's musical development.

Wolfgang Hildesheimer says of Mozart's first opera, written when he was 11: "His first *opera buffa, La finta semplice*, K. 51/46a, written before *Bastien und Bastienne*, between April and July 1768 in Vienna, is the work of an extraordinary child. His experience, musical and emotional, is not yet great enough for a masterpiece that would meet his later standards" (Hildesheimer, 1977, pp. 140, 141). And the critic John Stone (1990), after reviewing all of Mozart's known compositions, concluded: "While it is true that there are flashes of inspiration in many of the earlier works, probably the first which has a firm footing in the modern repertoire is the 'little' G Minor Symphony, K. 183, written when he was seventeen" (cited by Landon, 1990, p. 392).

Mozart was therefore not an exception to the ten-year rule, and he was no exception either in terms of the amount of effort that went into his development. What is true, of course, is that, having achieved thorough mastery over his domain by 12 or 13, he soared to unheard-of heights, with unheard-of lift in his wings. The study of prodigies has not revealed so much as a hint about why Mozart took flight and so many others, whose mastery compares with his, never get off the flight deck.

9. Arouses Hostility and Ambivalence

It has been part of the prodigy tradition to arouse as much negative as positive feeling, sometimes more. Inasmuch as the original meaning of the term was not confined to children, and referred to omens and portents and other strange events, it is not surprising that the label prodigy has not necessarily been a welcome one; it was not in Mozart's time. The most common negative reactions to Mozart's astounding feats were disbelief, suspicion that they were somehow fake, accusations of unnatural or sacreligious involvements, and of course jealousy.

Mozart and his father inadvertently played into such negative reactions by being naive about the rough-and-tumble world of the professional musician. They tended to believe that what by most accounts was fairly typical backbiting, intrigue, and efforts to achieve competitive advantage for scarce opportunities, were the most base treacheries. As a child Mozart was received well in most of the great houses of Europe, but then he was touted as a "miracle." As time passed, the Mozarts were faced with increasing indifference or worse from those who controlled musical career opportunities (Schenk, 1955).

In spite of the genuine hostility and jealousy that Mozart aroused, the story told in the play *Amadeus* by Peter Shaffer of a death plot by Antonio Salieri is very farfetched. There is little evidence that Salieri or anyone else saw Mozart as a sufficiently serious threat to lead to a plan to murder him. Still, although exaggerated, the play does make the point that great talent, along with the personal qualities that sometimes accompany it, tend to generate strong animosities by those closest to the one whose talent they must confront. Mozart was no exception to this tendency, and his behavior toward other musicians generally exacerbated the problem (Marshall, 1985).

It must be added that Mozart did not arouse *only* negative reactions among fellow musicians and those whom he wished to impress. There are many examples of genuine recognition of his talent and awe at his achievements. Although the degree of recognition he received during his lifetime was not commensurate with the quality of work that he did, he was widely known and highly praised during much of his brief life.

Interpretations like those of Wolfgang Hildesheimer (1977) pointing to a callous, indifferent Viennese public being the primary cause of his demise are exaggerated at best, simply untrue at worst. The reasons for Mozart's early death are both more subtle and more mundane than Hildesheimer and others would contend, as Peter Davies (1989) points out in a recent book (see also the present volume, chapter 7). It is likely that recognition and reward contributed to a decline in his spirits during the final years, but hardly enough to account for his early death.

10. A Mixture of Child and Adult Qualities

For many prodigies, the focus on developing their talents is often accompanied by an overly protected environment. There are stories told about prodigies who were unable to tie their own shoes or cut their own meat, even as adults (Revesz, 1925; Ostwald, 1991). This tendency to pamper and protect may well contribute to the impression that prodigies do not make the transition to adulthood as completely as most others do. It was true in several of the cases I studied as well that parents continued to do some things for their offspring that other children take over as a matter of course. Certainly it was true of Mozart's life that he was excused from dealing with most of life's day-to-day problems, particularly during the years when he traveled with his family.

Contrasted with the tendency to arrest development is an equally strong impression of prodigies that their overall development proceeds at an accelerated pace, thus rendering them the equivalent of people with children's bodies and adult's minds (Feldman, 1986). Perhaps because of the popularity of the idea of IQ or general intelligence, we have tended to assume that the prodigy's development could not be limited to a specific talent area, but must bring along with it all other mental functions. As was discussed earlier, Mozart's talents were very focused in music.

Most prodigies, and certainly Mozart, tend to be rather single-purpose organisms, radically advanced within their areas of expertise, relatively typical otherwise (Feldman, 1986). This discrepancy between an extraordinary precocity and seeming maturity in music or art or dance or mathematics, and normal or even arrested development in other areas, has led to the impression of prodigies as being mixtures of children and adults. Based on my experience with several prodigies, the impression seems to be on the whole accurate.

But there is more to the child/adult mixture than simply an unevenness in development, even more than an exaggeration of this discrepancy as a result of parental overprotectiveness. A *genuine* childlike quality can sometimes be detected in the work of known cases of extreme talent; Albert Einstein, for example, seemed to maintain a childlike sense of wonder about the universe.

Among great talents, Mozart was one whose work is often described as having the purity and lightness of a child's emotions. This is not to say that Mozart's music showed no development over time. There is no doubt that the 10- or 12-year-old prodigy, however impressive his work was, could not create the sustained, coherent, unique qualities that mark a composition as undeniably that of the mature Mozart. And one of the most distinctive features of a Mozart signature work is the incredible lightness and purity of emotion of a child, balanced perfectly against the deep wisdom that only comes from experience.

CONCLUSION: MOZART AS PRODIGY

The foregoing discussion should leave no doubt that Mozart in many ways resembled other prodigies, particularly in the focus of his talent, the extraordinary mastery of a domain at a very early age, the tendency to arouse both strong positive and negative emotions, the deep sense of inner confidence, and a set of people around him determined to bring forth his potential, ready and willing to stay the course and secure the resources essential to the process.

Less marked in Mozart's life were a long family history in music, an adolescent crisis in which one's competence seems to unravel, and a tendency to find prodigies among first-born males. Also unusual in Mozart's character was an exceptional sociability that may be unique among great prodigies.

Although these observations could not begin to explain how and why Mozart achieved the transcendent place he now holds among contributors to Western culture, they may help to comprehend better the nature of the prodigy in general, and the nature of the prodigy we know as Mozart in particular. Knowing this particular prodigy has been a difficult task, one made more difficult by a history of distortion of Mozart to fit this or that image. To conclude the present discussion, we will briefly consider the images of Mozart that must be transcended in order to actually know him.

MOZART AS ARTIFACT

The Idealized Mozart

During his nearly 36 years of life, Mozart enjoyed some major successes, if not full-blown triumphs, and also suffered some crushing disappointments. In some places (like Prague, for example), he was welcomed as a great man, while in others like his home town of Salzburg, his reputation never came close to matching his achievements. He died in Vienna amidst mixed prospects; had he survived the illness that beset him in the Fall of 1791, it is likely that he would have been able to sustain his fairly lavish life style, quite possibly even improve upon it (Solomon, 1983), but of course we will never know.

Within days of his death, the reality of Mozart quickly faded and the image-making began. As often happens, Mozart's place in the world of composition seemed to grow dramatically after he died. By the middle of the nineteenth century, the image of Mozart as a paragon of virtue, a perfect expression of the romantic ideal of the "genius," was more or less fully formed. A statue in Vienna's Burggarten behind the new Hofburg exemplifies the tendency to idealize Mozart, extending even to his unremarkable physical features. The statue could not possibly have used the real Mozart as its model.

In contrast with the idealized, Apollonian Mozart, the recent play *Amadeus* (Shaffer, 1982) gave us a Mozart who was little more than a savant, a boor who had no insight into his own talent nor the minimum of civility to find his way among his fellow beings. From Mozart as perfection itself, we found ourselves dealing with Mozart as buffoon: His gifts are inexplicable, a joke on humanity by a peevish God. In contrast to his self-anointed archrival, the devoted, civilized, professional Salieri, Mozart did nothing to earn his unearthly gifts, nor was he properly humble before their power (Marshall, 1985).

Of course neither image is accurate. Each serves as much to remind us of the preoccupations of a period in Western cultural history as it does of a portrait of a man. Each time such image-making occurs, it makes the task of learning who the real Mozart was a great deal more difficult. This, combined with the fact that the empirical evidence about Mozart's life is incomplete and occasionally virtually nonexistent, makes it unlikely that we will ever be able to know Wolfgang Mozart as he really was. For example, we have almost no information about Mozart's first four or five years in Salzburg and little about his earliest encounters with music; as a prodigy, information about early experience is utterly crucial, the moreso because the field is music. Music is perhaps the earliest talent to emerge of those that prodigies display, usually appearing between 2 and 6 years old (Feldman, 1986; Bamberger, 1992). By the time we begin to get information about Mozart's musical abilities and activities, his gift has already crystallized and taken form (Walters and Gardner, 1986).

The scholarly literature on Mozart's life and Mozart's music runs well into the hundreds, possibly the thousands of works. Each time a new fact is revealed or a more penetrating interpretation is offered than what was available, the cause of true understanding is advanced.

In the present discussion, the growing body of knowledge about prodigies was used as a template against which to compare the facts of Mozart's life. The aim of this exercise was not so much to force Mozart into a "prodigy mold" (as if that could be done), but to use what is known about prodigies as a base from which to gain a bit better view of this particular, this treasured prodigy.

The slow work of scholarship will always be done within a social, cultural context, and so will always be subject to limitations of perspective based on the influences of the moment. It is safe to say that the present discussion is no exception. Still, with time, we can hope to see some of the mists receding around the one we know as Mozart. It does nothing to diminish the greatness of his contributions to try to know him as he actually was rather than as the fulfillment of an image we need to create for him. In time perhaps we will know him better.

REFERENCES

Anderson, E., ed. (1966), *The Letters of Mozart and His Family.* New York: W. W. Norton.

Bamberger, J. (1982), Growing up prodigies: The midlife crisis. In: *Developmental Approaches to Giftedness and Creativity*, ed. D. H. Feldman. San Francisco, CA: Jossey-Bass, pp. 61–78.

—— (1992), *The Mind Behind the Musical Ear.* Cambridge, MA: Harvard University Press.

Baumgarten, F. (1930), *Wunderkinder psychologische unterschungen.* Leipzig: Johann Ambrosious Barth.

Bloom, B., ed. (1985), *Developing Talent in Young People.* New York: Ballantine Books.

Boyd, M. (1990), Who's who. In: *The Mozart Compendium: A Guide to Mozart's Life and Music*, ed. C. R. Landon. New York: Schirmer Books.

Davies, P. (1989), *Mozart in Person: His Character and Health.* Westport, CT: Greenwood Press.

Feldman, D. H. (1971), Map understanding as a possible crystallizer of cognitive structures. *Amer. Ed. Res. J.*, 8:485–501.

—— (1974), Universal to unique: A developmental approach to creativity. In: *Essays in Creativity*, ed. S. Rosner & L. Abt. Croton-on-Hudson, NY: North River Press.

—— (1986), *Nature's Gambit: Child Prodigies and the Development of Human Potential.* New York: Teachers College Press, 1991.

—— (1992), Mozart and the transformational imperative. Paper presented at the symposium: "Mozart and the Riddle of Creativity," sponsored by the Woodrow Wilson Center for Scholars, The Smithsonian Institution, Washington, DC, December.

Forman, M., director (1984), *Amadeus* (film). The Saul Zaentz Co.

Gardner, H. (1991), *The Unschooled Mind.* New York: Basic Books.

—— (1992), *How* unique is Mozart? Paper presented at the symposium: "Mozart and the Riddle of Creativity," sponsored by the Woodrow Wilson Center for Scholars, The Smithsonian Institution, Washington, DC, December.

Goldsmith, L. T. (1987), Girl prodigies. *Roeper Rev.*, 10:74–82.

Hayes, J. R. (1981), *The Complete Problem Solver.* Philadelphia: Franklin Institute Press.

Hildesheimer, W. (1977), *Mozart*, trans. M. Faber. New York: Vintage Books, 1983.

Howe, M. J. A. (1989), *Fragments of Genius.* London: Routledge & Kegan Paul.

Jahn, O. (1891), *Life of Mozart*, 3 vols., 2nd ed., trans. P. D. Townsend. London: Novello, Ewer.

Landon, C. R., ed. (1990), *The Mozart Compendium: A Guide to Mozart's Life and Music.* New York: Schirmer Books.

Lang, P. H., ed. (1963), *The Creative World of Mozart.* New York: W. W. Norton.

Marshall, R. L. (1985), Mozart/Amadeus: Amadeus/Mozart. *Brandeis Rev.,* 5:9–16.

Menuhin, Y. (1977), *Unfinished Journey.* New York: Alfred A. Knopf.

Nohl, L. (1893), *Mozart,* tr. J. J. Lalor. Chicago: A. C. McClurg.

Ostwald, P. (1991), *Vaslav Nijinsky: A Leap into Madness.* Secaucus, NJ: Lyle Stuart.

Pichler, K. (1844), *Denkwürdigkeiten aus meinem Leben,* ed. E. K. Blümml. Vienna, Munich, 1915.

Revesz, G. (1925), *The Psychology of a Musical Prodigy.* Freeport, NY: Books for Libraries Press, 1970.

Roberts, D. (1991), The real Amadeus. *Boston Globe Magazine,* January 13: pp. 18–23, 26.

Rolfe, L. M. (1978), *The Menuhins: A Family Odyssey.* San Francisco: Panjandrum/Aris Books.

Schenk, O. (1955), *Mozart and His Times,* tr. R. & C. Winston. New York: Alfred A. Knopf, 1960.

Shaffer, P. (1982), *Amadeus.* Harmondsworth, U.K.: Penguin.

Solomon, M. (1983), Review of W. Hildesheimer's *Mozart. Musical Quart.,* 69:270–279.

Stone, J. (1990), Reception. In: *The Mozart Compendium: A Guide to Mozart's Life and Work,* ed. C. R. Landon. New York: Schirmer Books.

Treffert, D. A. (1989), *Extraordinary People: Understanding "Idiot Savants."* New York: Harper & Row.

Walters, J., & Gardner, H. (1986), The crystallizing experience: Discovering an intellectual gift. In: *Conceptions of Giftedness,* ed. R. Sternberg & J. Davidson. New York: Cambridge University Press, pp. 306–331.

3

The Psychodynamics of Mozart's Family Relationships

Erna Schwerin, M.A.

Of the many Mozart studies that have appeared since his early death, only a very small number contain a probing and critically discerning viewpoint conducive to an understanding of the composer's personality, life style, and relationships with his family. I stated in my introduction to Peter Davies' study (1989) that every century has viewed Mozart differently by taking from him whatever suited contemporary needs. In the nineteenth and early twentieth centuries Mozart emerged as a stock roccoco figure, leading a charmed life. His music fulfilled a longing for a better world, and a personality to match had to be conjured up. Now twentieth-century sensibility is providing us with greater insight, enabling us to view him more realistically, albeit retrospectively, in the light of eighteenth-century mores.

In writing this paper I became aware of the need to resist the temptation of reducing Mozart's life story and interaction with his family to a case history. We know today that his pure creative greatness remained untouched by the negative aspects of his life. His detachment, that is, his ability to achieve a split of his ego between the extraneous circumstances of his existence and his creative work, accounts for this phenomenon. This was one of the very few areas in which he was able to move from the center (of his childhood) to the periphery, developing normal self-confidence, as contrasted with his fixation at an infantile level which accounted for the personality problems, and his functioning in more mundane aspects of living.

49

There is consensus that his father Leopold was the most significant figure in Mozart's life, although he was later replaced by Constanze (Schwerin, 1981) in important areas. As soon as Mozart's musical gifts became apparent at an early age, Leopold took complete charge of him. There is the story of mutual idealization ("Papa comes right after God"), and Leopold's tears when little Wolferl wrote a "concerto," or insisted on playing the violin without ever having had a lesson, with very few mistakes. There was then a relatively untroubled relationship between father and son. Mozart reported later that he was never punished by his father for his little transgressions or mischievous behavior; instead, his mother and the servants were blamed for any problems! (Schwerin, 1984). This set the stage early on for a sense of infantile omnipotence, strongly reinforced by Leopold, continuing later and affecting his self-discipline as Mozart had to move from the center to the periphery in significant areas of functioning as an adult. Still, the early encouragement and affirmation by the paternal figure were internalized by Wolfgang, enabling him to preserve his father's image as a human being, mentor, and teacher. Nannerl, too, had manifested considerable musical gifts early on, which were fostered actively by Leopold who instructed her in the clavier (Schwerin, 1985, 1986). Though he was deeply impressed by her talents and achievements, he transferred most of his attention to the five years younger son as soon as *his* gifts surfaced so dramatically. We will come back to the effects of this on Nannerl later on.

Some of Mozart's prominent character traits formed early did not undergo significant dynamic changes: Behaviorally, he retained his gregariousness and outgoing behavior and spontaneity; but the transformation of infantile narcissism into normal self-confidence seemed always to be limited to his sublime gifts as a composer and musician. In his personal relationships he had an almost insatiable affect hunger, needing to be loved and praised. When in his later years the pressures of daily living increased, and he had to cope with the frustrations of fruitless efforts for a position outside Salzburg and his father's recriminations and projections, his coping skills became adversely affected, and his high spirits were unconsciously placed in the service of denial to fight an underlying depression and narcissistic depletion.

Leopold became his son's entrepreneur during the early journeys (1762–1766) undertaken to present Wolfgang and Nannerl to the world (Schwerin, 1987). The father basked in the glory of the spreading fame of the youngsters. Wolfgang's promotion continued until his final departure from Salzburg in 1780, albeit indirectly, through contacts and correspondence. Early on, Leopold had trepidations about the children's fame not holding up once they entered adulthood. His preoccupation with this concern was an important factor in preventing Wolfgang's maturity; Leopold needed to preserve the image of the Wunderkind. In our time Leopold is often severely censured for the strenuous journeys undertaken at the children's early ages. I am not one of these detractors. It is not quite realistic to apply eighteenth-century mores of parental guidance to our standards of child rearing. What is often overlooked is that Leopold created an ambience conducive to stimulating optimal development of Mozart's prodigious gifts, and that his introduction to the world during childhood provided not only an arena for broadening the children's musical and cultural horizons, but set the stage for some of Mozart's future important and successful contacts and ventures. Leopold's influence on his son's emotional development is quite another matter. His motivations will become clearer when we take a look at the father's own personality and relate *his* familial history to his interaction with Wolfgang.

Intellectually, Leopold was a remarkable individual, whose authorship of the *Violinschule*, compositions, and musicological essays, had left their own imprint on his contemporaries *before* Mozart's birth. He was highly educated and his interests encompassed wide areas outside the realm of music. His own background made him vulnerable to the development of personality problems. He had left his native Augsburg for Salzburg at age 17, after his father's death. There had been problems with his brothers and mother. We can only assume that the loss of his father must have had a very strong effect on him, lacking as he was in maternal support. His mother was an unstable woman with character problems of paranoid proportions. The relative stability of Leopold's own character defenses derives from the fact that at the time of his father's death he must have already internalized some of the most crucial, positive aspects of the paternal bond. Leopold was strongly identified with the high educational standards his own father had projected for him, coupled with ambition and emphasis on high achievement; these Leopold adopted and integrated into a personality of predominantly obsessional traits. One may well ask the question, not previously raised in the literature on

Mozart, to what extent the loss of Leopold's own father may have played a crucial role in his excessive need to protect and control Wolfgang. It may, among other functions, have been in the service of mastery of his own experience, thus perpetuating Wolfgang's ineptness in handling his affairs, especially his finances, and in coping with situations of daily living (Schwerin, 1987). It is not in the least surprising that Mozart remained a child in this area, since everything was done for him until he moved to Vienna. Father and son were locked in a symbiotic relationship, in which they also acted out with each other complementary and similar attitudes. Sometimes Wolfgang "became" the father, when Leopold, finding himself in a position of helplessness and frustration, transferred the power of "life and death" (letter of July 13, 1778, to Wolfgang in Paris) to his son, begging him to return home to help support him and Nannerl (Anderson, 1966). I am referring here to the catastrophic journey to Paris and fruitless search for a position, followed by the mother's death. Leopold had felt that he could not trust Wolfgang to make this trip unaccompanied, and was himself unable to travel with him. The decision to designate mother as a chaperone was an astonishing one, coming from someone as rational as Leopold. He had hoped to find a way to ensure his continuing control of developments from afar by regular correspondence. But Anna Maria, while loved and respected by the family, was ill equipped to exercise any control over Mozart's movements; her compliant, passive personality was no match for her son's strong-willed rebellious one, of which she would experience ample proof during the extended journey. Mozart was a father's son. The mother had always been kept in the background during his childhood—it was Leopold who made all the domestic and musical decisions. Anna Maria adapted herself to them, undoubtedly not without some resentment. While she never lost her sense of humor, as reflected in her letters to Leopold, she also adjusted by a kind of stoicism. Still, her letters also bear witness to her health problems away from home, her loneliness, and complaints about being left on other occasions when Leopold and Nannerl joined Wolfgang in Munich for the premiere of his *La Finta giardiniera* in 1775.

Anna Maria had a musical heritage from her father. Schenk believes that it played a more important part in Mozart's own gifts than has been recognized in the literature. Musical talent of a quality and extent credited to *her* father has not been found in any of Mozart's other relatives. Although there is no direct evidence of any such gifts in Anna Maria herself, she was said to have had a natural talent for music and theatricals (Schenk, 1975). In her youth she was described as very beautiful, and at their wedding she and Leopold were referred to as the handsomest couple in Salzburg. Although the marriage had many positive features, as can be gleaned from the correspondence, the stresses of it were mostly caused by the idiosyncrasies of Leopold's very dominant, exacting personality. In order to minimize domestic strife, Anna Maria had to suppress any amount of self-assertion (Schwerin, 1984). Her sense of humor was of great help. Her letters resemble those of her son in their freshness and spontaneity, but they were much more staightforward than his. In contrast, Leopold's letters to his wife and son were demanding and censorious, especially those addressed to them when they were in Mannheim and Paris; Wolfgang's were evasive, placating, and often filled with trivia. Leopold exhorted his wife to read them before dispatch—it was the last straw—but she was powerless. Wolfgang did as he pleased, doing a great deal of socializing with the Webers and other friends. Anna Maria was longing for a return home; her privations were hard to bear and the subject of continual complaints in the correspondence. The family was in prolonged crisis. Surprisingly, we find very few references to Nannerl in Anna Maria's communications, despite the fact that the daughter's postscripts reflect a longing for the mother's presence. During the entire period of the mother's absence, only one letter addressed to Nannerl personally is documented, containing comments on Paris fashions! The situation with Wolfgang and her own concerns about health, comfort, and the future seemed at least for the moment to supersede all other considerations for Anna Maria.

But the mother's hopes of returning to Salzburg from Mannheim while the weather still permitted travel were dashed by Wolfgang's unsettled affairs and his strong resistance to leaving; Anna Maria's strong sense of obligation finally motivated her to accompany him; she barely coped with all the details alone—he was simply not available, but escaped to the comforts of the Webers. The close attachment he had formed to this family as a result of his love for the daughter Aloysia made a separation extremely difficult for him. He had also aroused Leopold's jealous anger by his frequent references to Herr Weber's positive character traits. When they finally left, it turned out that Anna Maria had not underestimated the ordeals of the journey, and the still greater hardships awaiting mother and son in Paris. The rest is history. This time Wolfgang's absences from the dingy quarters he and his mother occupied were more frequent and necessary than in Mannheim because he needed to look for commissions, pupils, and time to compose. Only the hope of returning home sustained Anna Maria. She developed illnesses intermittently, ultimately succumbing to what Peter Davies (1989) believes may have been a louse-born epidemic typhus fever (p. 49), on July 3, 1778, at age 57.

Some recent authors are divided about what Mozart was presumed to have felt at the time of his mother's death. Hildesheimer (1977) believes that it was "not an object loss, as we know of no manifestations of love such as towards his father." Ortheil (1982) puts Mozart's need to deny guilt as superseding all other feelings at that moment, citing his reference to her death as "inevitable . . . because of God's will" in the letter to Leopold of July 31, 1778. There is little doubt that Mozart felt guilt about his mother's death—a normal feeling under the circumstances, but we strongly disagree with Hildesheimer. Solomon's perceptive review (1983) of that author's book reinforces my belief that Mozart was much affected by the loss of his mother. Solomon aptly observes that Anna Maria did not make the demands on her son that his father did, allowing Mozart to take her love for granted. It is obvious that his father's love was essentially conditional in his demands for complete compliance and superior performance. The warmth and naturalness of Mozart's relationship with his mother is on record in the many letters the young Mozart addressed to her on his early travels. The unusual circumstances brought about by the journey, characterized by often burdensome togetherness, was atypical and would not have had a lasting effect on Mozart's feelings for her. Mozart's letter to his father of July 9, 1778, does reflect pain and grief most poignantly, and he must have felt it intensely. In addition to comforting his father and sister, he also had to comfort and orient himself in the present. Of course, he feared his father's recriminations, which were not long in coming. Specifically, Leopold blamed Wolfgang for belated medical attention; but viewed from today's viewpoint, medical incompetence, eighteenth-century style, would be a more apt description of the situation. Mozart had shown concern as his mother's health declined. He did not call on his pupils but stayed with her throughout the last weeks of illness; neither did he compose. It is really impossible to know if she could have been saved under any conditions in Paris.

Actually it was Leopold who had to confront his own guilt, and he projected it at least to some degree on Wolfgang. In the course of his wife's and son's absence he must have become increasingly aware of how unsound his decision about their journey together had been. It was the irony of fate that ultimately Mozart should have been left alone after all in a strange country, a situation which Leopold wanted to avoid at all costs, and for which the price turned out to be very high indeed. It is to Nannerl's everlasting credit that she did not blame her brother, so that their relationship remained harmonious after his return from Paris (Schwerin, 1985, 1986). He delayed his return for almost four months by various stopovers, some still in hope of escaping from Salzburg by securing a post elsewhere. This did not happen. When he finally arrived in his native city, he was accompanied by Bäsle (his cousin) whom he had invited to Munich and whom uncle Leopold had generously invited to Salzburg to please Wolfgang and, perhaps, to dilute the discomfort of the first meeting after the family's catastrophe. Wolfgang needed diversion badly—he had just been rejected as a suitor by Aloysia who in the interim had become a famous singer and no longer needed Mozart. It well-nigh broke his heart but he bravely coped in his typical mode of escape.

He seemed resigned to settle in Salzburg, reinstated by the archbishop with more favorable conditions. But a welcome commission from Munich to compose *Idomeneo* was to change all that. Wolfgang never returned to Salzburg from Vienna, where he had gone at the archbishop's request, and broke with him after a heated dispute. Leopold's long letters, his pleas, and threats designed to create more guilt, proved fruitless; Mozart remained adamant that he would fashion a freelance career in Vienna. It was clear that his return to Salzburg was only to appease his father and sister, and that his resignation finally had to give way to continued rebellion, especially after the heady success of his opera. Dynamically, Mozart's abandonment of his father was also a repetition of Leopold's departure from *his* family at a time when Leopold had been expected to take an active role in providing them with emotional (although not financial) support. He was the eldest son.

In Vienna it was again the Weber family that provided a home for Mozart. Father Weber had died. Mozart developed an attachment to Constanze, Aloysia's younger sister, fancying himself in love with her. I believe that his unconscious motivation was a strong identification with her as a victim of rejection by important others. Early on the Weber family had been persecuted by a feudal lord, forcing them to leave their hometown. Mozart must have received a full account of this situation earlier in Mannheim. He saw himself as Constanze's protector and rescuer even before he married her, and also unconsciously identified her with the heroine of the *Entführung*, the opera in progress just then. Certain parallels do exist: The name, whether chosen intentionally is difficult to say, the virtual "enslavement" by her mother, from whom he, like Belmonte, must rescue her after a long struggle, which was also a premarital scenario, directed and enacted by Frau Weber. The marriage brought about the fulfillment of Mozart's rescue fantasy which, in addition, contained elements of his own experience with the archbishop. In other respects, Mozart's attitude toward Constanze offered a strong parallel to that of Leopold toward him: He frequently adopted the same moralizing stance toward his wife. Another holdover from the past was Mozart's overconcern and solicitude toward Constanze about her health. It is reasonable to assume that some of his guilt about his mother's death played a part in producing this need (Schwerin, 1981).

The marriage, which took place prior to the arrival of Leopold's consent and over his strong objections, did offer certain gratifications. It is questionable that Constanze was in love with Wolfgang. She had welcomed, and responded to, his attentions, and was not averse to becoming a wife of a promising composer and artist. In later years, after Mozart's death, she described her relationship with him in terms of *being* loved rather than loving. She also relished the unaccustomed gratification of being looked after and cherished, as well as the domestic comforts. But as the years passed she began to feel stifled, looking for escapes. Her six pregnancies were indeed debilitating. She began to take frequent cures in a nearby spa, leaving Mozart increasingly to his own devices, sometimes for prolonged periods, although he joined her whenever he could. Some of Mozart's biographers are strongly critical of Constanze's absences, and although Mozart was particularly sensitive to separations he tolerated them, missing her sorely, as he did during his own travels. He wrote her daily notes, making up pet names for her, and other endearments, even when they were together. According to some writers, Mozart and Constanze supposedly were at times unfaithful to each other. We really do not know of any concrete situations or reliable sources for these inferences, nor of any disagreements or crises in the marriage. From what has been inferred, the attachment was a result of unresolved early problems, as well as sexual attraction. Mozart's need for his wife seemed to be emotionally stronger than hers for him—had he not replaced his father with her as much as this was possible? One noteworthy feature of Constanze's adaptation to the marriage was her tendency to overidentify with Mozart's needs and decisions, mostly in financial matters. It was he who spent money freely and lavishly, but she has been blamed for laxness in handling domestic matters. In actuality we know now that she only went along with *his* spending habits (Schwerin, 1981).

The couple paid one visit to Salzburg in 1783. Mozart had postponed it as long as he could. After all, Leopold and Nannerl had denied Constanze the friendship and acceptance which she had so fervently sought. Nannerl's entries in her diary reflect the mutual activities in very concrete terms, but we can infer that a friendly hospitality was extended to the young couple. There was a quasi-reconciliation in 1785 when Leopold visited Vienna, witnessing some of his son's most dramatic successes as a composer of the piano concertos and quartets dedicated to Haydn, as well as the emperor's recognition at a performance. He also could not help but admire Constanze's ability to manage the household finances.

We have saved Nannerl's role (Schwerin, 1985, 1986) in the family's scenario for the last. Let us go back for a moment to look at her vis-à-vis Wolfgang as a child. A beautiful, gifted youngster, Leopold had begun teaching her at age 7. Wolfgang, five years younger, became a keen observer of her lessons, beginning to imitate her at an early age. Nannerl would later remember her childhood up to adolescence as the happiest period of her life. Though regimented, she and her brother enjoyed carefree times in each other's company with deep mutual affection, and both relished Nannerl's own special fame as a performer on the piano. Before Wolfgang's extraordinary gifts had become apparent, she had indeed been the apple of her father's eye, but had to take second place when he began concentrating on her brother's genius. Still, there is no evidence of any unusual sibling rivalry in childhood. On the journeys she was not heard as a soloist in every city, but when presented she played the most difficult sonatas and concertos with the greatest ease and adult musical taste. Leopold called her "one of the most accomplished pianists in Europe" at age 12 (Schenk, 1975). She was highly acclaimed not only by the public but also by Wolfgang. Taking all this in her stride with an appealing modesty, she told her admirers: "I am only my brother's pupil!" Musical rivalry did not exist between brother and sister either; each adored the other's performances, with Wolfgang surpassing

Nannerl only in improvisation and composition, although he was un-
questionably the star attraction. Nannerl's happiest and proudest moments were attached to these journeys. In later years she would have
to settle for remaining on the sidelines, in the shadow of her brother's
fame. From 1769 on she no longer had the opportunity to present
herself in public. At age 18 she would have been sufficiently mature
as an artist to define herself, had she wanted a career as a pianist. It
is very doubtful that such a possibility was ever considered by her
parents; if it existed for her, it would have had to remain an illusion.
There is no record of discussions, plans, or of her own thoughts on
the subject.

The warm, affectionate relationship between brother and sister is
documented in the lively, detailed correspondence during Wolfgang's
absences from Salzburg; he teased her lovingly, sometimes wrote in
Italian. He also composed several works for her, including the *Diverti-
mento* K. 251 (1776), the *Sonata for Four Hands*, K. 381 (1783), and the
Concerto for Two Pianos, K. 365 (1779). In 1770 Nannerl had presented
herself as a composer for the first time with a song. Wolfgang, expressing surprise and pleasure, called it "beautiful." They also ex-
changed compositions by other composers, and Wolfgang added "instructions" for performance.

Nannerl suffered acutely from her brother's and mother's departure in 1777. She took to her bed with a severe headache and gastroin-
testinal symptoms, associated with strong feelings of separation and
loss. Nannerl, like her mother, had difficulty handling negative feelings about separation; both had in common a tendency to express
them through their body. Her mother's absence completely changed
Nannerl's life. Not only did she have to cope with taking charge
of the household, but the relationship with her father underwent
significant changes; the mutual dependency and interaction with the
family was no longer as diluted as before, so that the closeness between
father and daughter increased. The outlook for her own future, however, was bleak; Leopold counted on her continued presence in the
home, and she, too, felt an obligation to comply. Although several
young men competed for Nannerl's hand, and she had fallen in love
with one of them, she seemed resigned to her fate of remaining single.
Leopold had found fault with all her suitors, ostensibly for economic
reasons. Perhaps for the first time she may have envied her brother
for his freedom of choice in marriage. She may even have projected
her negative feelings on Mozart's bride, denying her friendship and

acceptance. She filled her time with looking after the household, supervising the servants, and took much pleasure and comfort in teaching piano, a task at which she excelled and, unlike her brother, also enjoyed. It was later said that a pupil of Nannerl's could be easily recognized by the precision of performance. When she finally married an elderly aristocrat with five children and moved to nearby St. Gilgen in 1784, Leopold was resigned to remaining alone. He had consented to the marriage, which was one of convenience, because Nannerl was 33 years old and he feared for her future after his death. They kept in close touch by correspondence (there were almost daily long letters from him), visiting from time to time. When Nannerl gave birth to a boy, named Leopold, the baby was left with the grandfather. The decision to separate from her first and only natural child was indeed a puzzling one on Nannerl's part. I suspect that the rearing of five stepchildren, some of whom were described to have been very difficult, played an important part in her motivation.

The correspondence between Mozart and his father had diminished after his move to Vienna, and none of Leopold's letters after 1781 are extant, though they are known to have existed. Wolfgang rarely wrote to his sister after her marriage—there is a large gap in the correspondence between 1784 and 1787, the year of Leopold's death, when there was again a brief contact regarding the disposition of the estate. A dispute had developed between them about this matter, leading to a breach which was never healed. Mozart never revealed his financial struggles and his intermittent illnesses to his sister. After his death, she was stunned and deeply saddened to learn about her brother's plight.

Leopold's death at age 68 in 1787 affected Mozart deeply. He had written a touching and consoling letter to him during his illness, but learned too late about his death to attend the funeral. I agree with Langegger (1978) that an important part of Mozart's self ceased to exist after his father's death. For Nannerl, too, Leopold's passing caused a deep and lasting bereavement. A notation on a bundle of letters, stemming from her later life, reads: "Looked over in 1803."

In closing, let me inject a cautionary note: Mozart was and is a gift to all humanity. Regardless of the new vistas which have opened up in recent times for a better understanding of him, we always need to remind ourselves that genius can never be lured into predictability, and that certain facets of Mozart's life and personality must ever elude us.

REFERENCES

Anderson, E., ed. (1966), *The Letters of Mozart and His Family*. New York: W. W. Norton.

Davies, P. J. (1989), *Mozart in Person. His Personality and Health*. Westport, CT: Greenwood Press.

Deutsch, O. E. (1961), *Mozart. Die Dokumente seines Lebens*. Kassel: Bärenreiter.

Hildesheimer, W. (1977), *Mozart*. Frankfurt am Main: Suhrkamp.

Langegger, F. (1978), *Mozart. Vater und Sohn. Eine psychologische Untersuchung*. Zurich: Atlantis.

Mozart, W. A. (1962), *Briefe und Aufzeichnungen*. Kassel: Bärenreiter.

Ortheil, H.-J. (1982), *Mozart in Innern seiner Sprachen*. Frankfurt: Collection S. Fischer.

Schenk, E. (1975), *Mozart. Eine Biographie* (paperback). Goldmann Verlag.

Schwerin, E. (1981), *Constanze Mozart. Woman and Wife of a Genius*. New York: Friends of Mozart, Inc.

—— (1984), Anna Maria Mozart. A profile of Mozart's mother. *Newsletter No. 16*. New York: Friends of Mozart, Inc.

—— (1985), Maria Anna ("Nannerl") Mozart. A profile of Mozart's sister. *Newsletter No. 19* (Fall). New York: Friends of Mozart, Inc.

—— (1986), Maria Anna ("Nannerl") Mozart. A profile of Mozart's sister. *Newsletter 20* (Spring). New York: Friends of Mozart, Inc.

—— (1987), Leopold Mozart. Profile of a personality. New York: Friends of Mozart, Inc.

—— (1989), Introduction. In: *Mozart in Person: His Personality and Health*, by P. J. Davies. Westport, CT: Greenwood Press.

Solomon, M. (1983), Review of *Mozart* (1977) by W. Hildesheimer. *Musical Quart.*, Spring: pp. 270–279. Frankfurt am Main: Suhrkamp.

All newsletters and monographs published by the Friends of Mozart are available *only* to members of the organization.

4

Mozart and Secular Awe: Our Need for Genius in an Age of Uncertainty

Leonard S. Zegans, M.D.

Imagine the scene in a carriage conveying Mozart out of Paris after his disastrous trip there with his mother. His great expectations after joyously bidding his father and Salzburg goodbye (to say nothing of the Archbishop) were completely dashed; he had received vague promises, useless second-hand watches, waited for bored aristocrats in drafty drawing rooms, and was regarded by many as an arrogant, faded prodigy. He was not petted, courted, and flattered. And to add to his despair when his mother died, he could not bring himself to write the news to his father. As the gates of Paris closed behind him, we can only begin to imagine his thoughts of the prospect of being trapped again in Salzburg with his father and Archbishop Colloredo, writing weekly church masses. He picks up a pen, opens his writing tablet, sighs, and pens a letter to his father.

My Dear Papa,

You have no idea what a secret triumph this trip has been. Everywhere musicians of discernment have praised my works. True, I have not received many commissions and no position as Kapellmeister has materialized. I have been cold, neglected, and worst of all, Mamma has died. There have been scandalous rumors about me and I have been disappointed in love. You might ask what is there to be happy about? And rightly you may inquire. Yet, I had a vision as the coach was leaving Paris about what lies

61

ahead many years in the future. This will be hard to believe Papa, yet I am convinced that it is true. I envisioned that my face will be printed on shirts sold in the foyers of concert halls all over the world. For some reason they are called T-shirts. Perhaps people will wear them when they imbibe the popular Indian infusion and eat delicious finger cakes. I also had a premonition that year in and year out concerts would be held in my honor with such strange names as *Mostly Mozart, Midsummer-Mozart, Midwinter Mozart* but unfortunately nothing indicates similar festivals held in the Autumn and Spring. People will listen to my music in their homes by merely pushing a button, and invisible singers and musicians will fill their chambers with my music. I know that you will contend that the strains of events, combined with a little too much snuff and the lack of air in the coach have addled my brain. Yet, I assure you that these things will happen. What is more, people will sit in darkened theaters and watch magic lantern shows of my life. They will even see you, but only briefly, and for some reason come to believe that Signor Salieri wishes to poison me out of jealousy for my talent. A Swiss writer named Hesse will write a novel in which I fly through the heavens with a strange character called Steppenwolf clinging to my pigtail and some mad Irish playwright named Shaw will set characters in an opera that I have only dreamed of writing on stage conversing with the Devil. Yes, Yes, you will say that it is clear that all your worries about me are justified and if only I would confine myself to writing German marches and pious church music all would be well. I know that I have been a disappointment to you lately but I think that I have a fairly realistic notion of my worth. Oh incidentally, on my travels in Mannheim I met a wonderful family named Weber. I think that I will marry one of the daughters, her name is Aloysia. You will love her, and well you may ask how I can be sure she will be my bride? Well, my dreams have showed me I will be successful and have this beautiful angel Weber besides me as my sweetly singing bird. Despair not Papa, there are strange and wonderful things that lie ahead, the future is amazing and not grim. I know Papa that you don't think that I am ever serious but am silly and frivolous. I know that I have wonderful music inside of me and that I must be free to write it and that only people who are free themselves or wish to be can be moved by it. So back to Salzburg.

Your Wolfie.

Now of course fathers are often skeptical of their sons' ambitions and fantasies of their future. A nice, secure position in a city like Augsburg would have satisfied Leopold for his son. There would be fine chamber sessions with the Landgraf and Gräfin or what have you, pale little countesses taking pianoforte lessons, and of course subscription concerts. For Papa Mozart too much talent could be a dangerous thing. And yet if this watchful father had had his way and if Wolfgang had been a dutiful son, why then we would not have *our* Amadeus. It is very clear by virtue of the fact that we have celebrated the death of a not-very-popular eighteenth-century Viennese composer who was buried in an unmarked grave that we have a great need for Mozart. Yes, we love his music, but he has become much more than that, he has become a needed cultural icon, indeed a secular saint. "The genius, as previously the saint, has direct access to truth by an invisible and unexplained route, while the person of talent must use regular and repeatable methods to find his way forward step by step, rather than by a singular flash of insight. A genius arrives at truth by grace, and not by works" (Hampshire, 1991).

In past centuries there was a special place for men and women who heard the inner harmony of the cosmos; who had glimpses of something beyond the daily struggle for survival, power, and instantaneous moments of pleasure. Humankind has always had a yearning for those messengers who went beyond the mundaneness of everyday life to tell us that there was a sweetness, an order, a restoring grace to the universe. Those voices, whether of the Buddha, Isaiah, Jesus, Julian of Norwich, St. Francis, or Meister Eckhart have faded since the rise of the scientific revolution. As our existentialist writers tell us, we appear trapped with No Exit in a silent and seemingly cold universe. We still tell the old stories of the burning bush, of the ride to Damascus, of the turning of water into wine, but we have come to see them as pictures in a Sunday school book and not as living realities. Yet there are some humans whom we believe have been touched by a special gift to lift our spirits and make us believe in something sublime beyond ourselves. It is something which is more than beauty, it is an awe of a universe that is yet accessible to our understanding. We romanticize these geniuses, and come to see them often as secular martyrs, misunderstood, and often driven mad by their visions. Certainly Van Gogh has played such a role as the archetype of the artist as possessed visionary. His paintings have surpassed the realm of art as an object and have become relics of this secular awe.

And what of Mozart, that musical stenographer of *God's* melodies as the Salieri figure in *Amadeus* would have it. As Ludwig Wittgenstein said to Bertrand Russell "Beethoven and Mozart are the sons of God" (Hampshire, 1991). There is a popular feeling that Mozart's music is "cheerful," "gay," filled with "mirth" and "joy." Yet, of course, there is something more, an overcoming of despair, a sense of forgiveness, an acceptance of the vanity, lust, and self-deceptions of people. Mozart tells us that everybody does these things, it is part of the human condition, and we are no less deserving of love for our follies. Yet what cannot be forgiven is pomposity, cruelty, and vulgarity. We need Mozart because he did not lose his humanity and enjoyment of life in the face of all the insults and disappointments and because he mixed the music of the spheres with the melodies of humankind. Somehow even his characters who march off to war never reach the battlefields, but like Cherubino, stay to make love instead.

We must not think of Mozart as a "naif," "a bubbling innocent"; he saw and experienced too much of the dark side of life. Yet he did not let it define him or his music. He assimilated it into his works giving them depth and profundity, but retaining always the wonder of the child, the sense of spontaneity and play. So at night when we are worn down by talk of riots, recession, and oil slicks we do ourselves the favor of listening to Mozart as did the Army doctor in *M.A.S.H.* who found sanity in the *Clarinet Concerto* after tending to the wounded and dying. We need our Mozart to help us sense something of the cosmos but also to root us securely here on earth, in our own lives. He does us the favor of bestowing the fruits of his genius, we must return that favor by never making him into an unchanging icon or worse still a commodity.

Our culture tends to regard the genius as a mystery, a being specially blessed and often wounded because of his unique gifts. He is the heir to the mythical being Philoctetes, who was given the special gift of having a bow that would always find its mark, but who paid the price of suffering from an ever-suppurating wound. We are also inclined to see geniuses as separate beings not really related to the time and culture in which they live. They are seen as passing through their society often ignored or misunderstood, only to be "discovered" by later generations.

Yet geniuses are indeed flesh and blood individuals with parents, friends, spouses, lovers, publishers, teachers, enemies, and patrons. They undeniably have remarkable intellectual capacities and special perceptive sensibilities. But the flowering of their talent requires a setting, an environment which can help bring their prodigal abilities to a concrete realization. They are also more than stenographers of God; they work hard, select their projects with care, and have the courage to present their work for public appraisal. So using Mozart as our model, how well does he reflect some of the assumptions of contemporary scholars about what is required to turn prodigious talent into mature genius? They most often possess:

1. *A high general intelligence and exceptional specific abilities.* Gifted individuals tend to have relatively high levels of general intelligence and extremely high levels of abilities in the fields of their expertise.

2. *An exceptional capitalization upon patterns of abilities.* The gifted not only have high levels of general and specific abilities, but seem to have a capacity for making the most of what abilities they have. The gifted seem particularly well able to bring their strengths to bear upon their domain of expertise and to find ways of compensating for their relative deficiencies in other areas.

3. *Exceptional environmental shaping abilities.* Exceptional individuals seem to be able to capitalize upon their environments with much the same flair with which they capitalize upon their abilities. When the environment does not suit them, they mold rather than succumb to it, and often end up shaping it for others as well as for themselves.

4. *An exceptional problem-finding ability.* The gifted are individuals who are able to find problems that are large in scope, important in the context of the field, and tractable in terms of being operationally studied or acted upon.

5. *An exceptional ability to conceive higher order relations.* They view their work not only as a series of isolated or loosely related projects, but as part of an evolving master plan or system that they create over time. Their life's work often reveals a kind of unity and systematization that is lacking in the work of the less gifted.

6. *An exceptional environment which has role models, teachers, and sensitive critics.* The gifted must have mentors and a critical environment that will nurture their particular talent. The individual whose potential expertise is in a more highly valued domain of endeavor is likely to be better recognized than is the individual whose potential experience is in a field that, even if recognized, is accorded less value. (These categories reflect the ideas of Sternberg and Davidson [1983].)

7. *An exceptional ability to retain self-confidence and belief in the value of the work in the face of social rejection and isolation.* Often as the genius moves into new and adventurous realms of creativity the support that may have been present earlier in his career is withdrawn. There is need of an inner strength to sustain their work and present it publicly in the absence of praise and general understanding.

Creative work is part of an evolving life project that is embedded in the cultural and intellectual context of the individual's existence. Mozart lived at a certain time, was exposed to a particular family with its unique advantages and stresses. He lived in a country that valued music, but of certain styles and convictions. He had certain resources and opportunities made available to him, but lacked many others. Mozart selected certain elements from his life and discarded others to create music that both looked back to his past and saw far ahead into an uncharted future. In this volume we examine the life of Mozart with some of these ideas in mind and see how he was able to take his abundant talents and mold them into works of unique genius. Perhaps even the passing of his mother, the failures of Paris, and the dread of long winters with the Archbishop and Papa helped to shape a young man of immense talent into an adult who could confront the pleasures and perils of genius, and become an artist of unsurpassed creativity.

It was George Balanchine, I believe, who once said that there was nothing that Mozart ever wrote that couldn't be put to dance. If there is a Dance of Life then Mozart indeed becomes its Kapellmeister.

REFERENCES

Hampshire, S. (1991), A review of *Ludwig Wittgenstein: The Duty of Genius* by R. Monk. *NY Rev. Books*, 38/3:3–6.
Sternberg, R. J., & Davidson, J. E. (1983), Insight in the gifted. *Ed. Psychologist*, 18:51–57.

5

Wolfgang's Wobbly Self-Worth

Gary S. Gelber, M.D.

Could Mozart, one of the greatest musical geniuses, have had wobbly self-worth? This discussion will be concerned with Mozart's self-worth during the first two-thirds of his short life, that is, until he was about 23 years old. To my knowledge, this subject has not been addressed in the literature on Mozart. The focus will be on Mozart's feelings of self-worth to the exclusion of other aspects of his multifaceted personality.

I was surprised when I discovered Mozart's self-references, because I did not expect a person of such great talent to possess the characteristics which I uncovered in my study of his letters. This article will relate what Mozart reveals about himself through his own writings, for which Emily Anderson's translation of the letters of Mozart and his family (Anderson, 1966) was my primary source.

Although he was a great musical genius, Mozart's feelings about himself reflected other aspects of his life experience and of his personality. Most important among these were his appearance, his father Leopold's assessment of him, and his own conception of himself as a person functioning in society, apart from his musical talent.

Mozart was not a handsome man. He was "small, thin, pale in colour, and entirely lacking in any pretensions as to physiognomy and bodily appearance" (Deutsch, 1966, p. 462). He had a soft voice. Mozart's sister wrote that he was "handsome . . . as a child. It was

Acknowledgments. I would like to thank Erna Schwerin for her help and for translating Mozart's difficult language.

only after the small-pox [at age 11] that he became so disfigured . . ."
(Deutsch, 1966, p. 493). He had a "malformed left external ear" (Davies, 1989, p. 2).

We know that children compare themselves competitively with
members of their own families. Mozart's comparison of his appearance with that of his parents, who were "the handsomest couple in
Salzburg," and with his sister, "a regular beauty," must have affected
his feelings of self-worth (Deutsch, 1966, p. 462).

Mozart's letters allow us to glimpse some of his thoughts about
life and about himself. Mozart portrayed himself in a negative manner
in some of his letters. For example, in a letter to his sister which he
sent home from Milan, the 14-year-old Mozart wrote: "to my sister I
send a pockmark of a kiss and I remain the same old . . . old
what? . . . the same old buffoon" (Anderson, 1966, p. 113).

Mozart's letter is relevant to the issue of his self-disparagement
in two ways. First, he refers to himself in a compromised way—as a
"buffoon." Second, he reveals his sensitivity to the effects of smallpox
on his face. It is as if the pox were so prevalent in him, that even his
kisses could have their own pockmarks. Mozart's joke suggests that
his kiss could contaminate her skin and, in doing so, could render
her appearance more equal to his own pockmarked appearance.

The same tendency to devalue this beautiful sister's appearance
is illustrated in Mozart's letter from the following week. Mozart sent
his sister "a hundred kisses or smacks on your marvellous horse face"
(Anderson, 1966, p. 115). Another joke, but in this one there is a
playful devaluation of her appearance by comparing her face to that
of a horse. If Mozart, in his humor, could pockmark his sister with a
kiss, or have her take on a horselike appearance, perhaps she might
not outshine him quite so much

Later in his life Mozart showed great sympathy toward people
who had disfigurements. For example, after he visited a composer
who was disfigured by syphilis, he wrote the following: "his appearance . . . so wrung my heart that all I could say half sobbing was: 'With
my whole heart I pity you. . . .' (I was so distracted and trembled so
in every limb that I could hardly speak.)" (p. 303).

Not only did Mozart on occasion refer to himself as a "buffoon,"
he also referred to himself in other compromised ways. In a letter
written two months later to his mother and sister, Mozart wrote, "I
am a fool as everyone knows" (p. 128).

Later in his fourteenth year he wrote to his mother and sister: "I am your Simple Simon of a son and Jack Pudding of a brother" (p. 145). The "Jack Pudding" reference was to a clown in a marionette theater, something like the clown in a Punch and Judy Show: a boisterous, aggressive identity for Mozart.

After visiting St. Peter's Basilica in Rome when he was 14, he wrote to his mother and sister: "I have had the honour of kissing St. Peter's foot [the foot of the statue] . . . and as I have the misfortune to be so small, I, that same old dunce Wolfgang Mozart had to be lifted up" (p. 128). Mozart seemed to feel that his short stature was a "misfortune."

Mozart suggested in other ways that he had compromised feelings of self-worth. For example, he wrote, "My pen is not worth a fig nor is he who is holding it" (p. 150).

Mozart used animal imagery in referring to himself, and much of the imagery is unflattering. He compared himself to pigs—in particular, to the posterior of the pig. He compared his music writing to the urination of pigs: "[He] cannot write as I do, I mean, as sows piddle" (p. 110).

Over the years, Mozart described himself in ways that indicate feelings of compromised self-worth. To give a brief sample of this tendency, he referred to himself as a "fool" (p. 240), "dunce" (p. 128), "little" (p. 350), "very mediocre" (p. 350), "queerest of fishes" (p. 430), and "duffer" (p. 501).

Mozart's humor reveals aspects of his self-worth. Studies of jokes show that they can contain an inner meaning and personal truth (Freud, 1905, p. 208). Like a comedian whose jokes and jibes reveal issues that are personal and sometimes embarrassing, that would be difficult to reveal without the packaging of humor, so Mozart reveals important facets of his personality through his jokes about himself.

Mozart jokingly referred to himself as a "Pig's Tail" (Anderson, 1966, p. 653), and this comparison symbolizes one aspect of his devalued self-worth. Yet Mozart's writings also reveal a certain pride in his urinary and anal products. Mozart writes the following about himself in a poem from his twenty-second year:

"as long as he can fart,
As long as he can piddle and shit it with the best,
So long will he . . . be blest" (p. 430).

Defecation and musical composition were associated in his mind on a few occasions: "The concerto . . . I'll scribble . . . some day when I'm shitting" (p. 457). On one occasion Mozart linked the elaboration of a musical theme with anality: "I . . . played the theme over again, but this time arseways" (p. 339). He is referring to playing the theme backwards, i.e., "arseways." The context makes it clear that he was proud of his arseways improvisation. Mozart portrayed feelings of superior self-worth using anal expressions.

Mozart wrote compositions with anal titles and texts, for example, K. 233, *Leck mir den Arsch fein recht schön saube* (*Lick my arse nice and clean*). In his canon *Leck mich im Arsch* (K. 231/382c), the text is "Lick my arse, hurry" (Marshall, 1991, p. 147).

Mozart appears to have attempted to compensate for feelings of low self-worth with grandiose fantasies concerning his anal products. In a letter to his cousin, who was also his paramour, Mozart described himself as "a worthless cousin," but he also showed how he overvalued his products as well: "Blow into my behind. It's splendid food. May it do you good" (Anderson, 1966, pp. 651–652). With his anal imagery, Mozart routinely devalued others, as in the following written to the same cousin: "I shit on your nose and it will run down your chin" (p. 358).

Mozart, at age 21, clearly took great relish in writing the following to his father:

> I would like . . . [the following painted on the dart gun] targets. A short man with fair hair, shown bending over and displaying his bare arse. From his mouth come the words: "Good appetite for the meal." The other man to be shown booted and spurred with a red cloak and a fine fashionable wig. He must be of medium height and in such a position that he licks the other man's arse. From his mouth come the words: "Oh, there's nothing to beat it. So, please. If not this time, another time" [Anderson, 1966, pp. 357–358].

Mozart was a short man with fair hair. Mozart's father as well as Hieronymus Colloredo, the archbishop of Salzburg, could fit the description of the other man.

Mozart seems to have felt some concern that, without his fecal armaments, he would be depleted of resources. In a probable reference to his father, who had just accused him of lying, Mozart wrote:

"whoever doesn't believe me, may lick me. . . . [But] I fear that my muck will soon dry up and that he won't have enough if he wants to sup" (p. 501).

In these pen portraits, Mozart puts others into the position of worshiping his products. He manifests what we could call anal grandiosity. In doing so he achieves a fantasied revenge on them. By engaging in such maneuvers, Mozart could compensate for his sense of low self-worth. Mozart may have felt like a "Pig's Tail" (p. 653), but something admirable comes out of this "Tail."

The central issue is that Mozart, for all his lofty genius, lacked confidence in himself. He wrote about this subject when he was 21: "[A]s soon as people lose confidence in me, I am apt to lose confidence in myself" (p. 485). Mozart seemed to be saying that he relied on external sources for a feeling of self-worth.

Mozart also referred to himself as an elevated, superior person. At times, though, immediately after his reference to his elevated status, he depicted himself in a compromised or even humiliated manner. For example, when he was 21, writing in a letter to his father, Mozart made a reference to a great honor that the Pope had bestowed on him: the Order of the Golden Spur. Mozart signed his letter: "Wolfgang Amadé Mozart Knight of the Golden Spur and, as soon as I marry, of the Double Horn . . ." (p. 385). This was a reference to his expectation that he will be cuckolded, "as soon as I marry."

Why would a person of his talent think of making such references? I think that at various times he felt both proud and devalued, depending on the circumstances and on his mood.

His letters contain many such juxtapositions of elevated status and worth, followed immediately by a contrasting self-portrayal of low, devalued, or humiliated status. Mozart's feelings about himself tend to polarize. There is a dualism of superior and inferior self-worth. Such self-descriptions epitomize the polarities of Mozart's self-worth.

Musicians of the eighteenth century could be applauded enthusiastically by the aristocracy, yet they might enter the palace only through the back door, and take their meals with the servants. And Mozart had to deal with such treatment. But for Mozart, the polarities in his self-worth were pronounced and personal, and this resulted in his being easily vexed by indignities.

Yet Mozart had realistic and proud feelings regarding his great abilities as a musician. For example, when he was 22, he indicated his recognition of his "talent for composition . . . which God in his goodness has so richly endowed me (I may say so without conceit, for I feel it now more than ever)" (p. 468).

Even though Mozart did not apparently have doubts about himself as a composer, his self-disparaging statements show that he did have devalued notions about himself as a person. We have seen how Mozart's appearance may have contributed to a feeling of not being the equal of his handsome parents and beautiful sister. Mozart's relationship with his father was also important in contributing to his insecure sense of self-worth.

Those of us who love Mozart's music owe a debt of gratitude to his father, Leopold Mozart, for his assiduous attention to his son's musical and general education. Leopold was an extraordinarily devoted, attentive father. Mozart's mother was of course important as well to his development. But for the purposes of this discussion, we will focus only on Leopold because he appears to have had more of a negative influence on Mozart's self-worth.

A Wunderkind can bring out strong old longings as well as new wishes and needs in the parent (Levinger, 1979, p. 332). Leopold turned to his son to find vicarious gratification for his own need for worth and achievement, and he strove to satisfy his grandiose longings.

Leopold wrote to 22-year-old Mozart: "from you I have expected all" (Anderson, 1966, p. 491). And we can take Leopold's statement at face value: He did expect "all" from his Wunderkind possession. Leopold did not differentiate enough between his own aims and accomplishments, and those of his son.

Leopold had a " 'til death do us part" expectation of his son. Leopold indicated that Wolfgang should not have romantic interests, should not make decisions for himself, and should not be independent. Leopold wanted Wolfgang to be the family breadwinner.

Schwerin (1987) stated: "So long as Wolfgang was a Wunderkind Leopold could revel in, and identify with, the narcissistic gratifications of success. But constant fears of the future haunted him after Wolfgang's adolescence, . . ." (p. 19). Leopold attempted to put a boa constrictor hold on Wolfgang: "you really must consider first of all the welfare of your parents, or else your soul will go to the devil," Leopold wrote his 22-year-old son (Anderson, 1966, p. 480). When Wolfgang did not fulfill Leopold's egocentric plans, his condemnations of Wolfgang were crushing: "what a lot I have had to swallow on your account. The Prince's conduct can only bend me, but yours can crush me. He can only make me ill, but you can kill me," the father wrote (p. 491).

Such criticisms could well lead to feelings of low self-worth in the most gifted child. As early as age 14, Mozart noted that "Papa wrote such cutting remarks . . ." (p. 172). Leopold's hypercritical manner probably went back many years in Mozart's life and preceded Mozart's adolescent attempts to free himself from his father's control.

Leopold even criticized his son's musical compositions: "I have not given any of your symphonies to be copied, because I suspect that when you are older and have more insights, you will be glad that no one got hold of them . . ." (p. 619).

In his letters, Mozart's self-devaluation often occurred after his father attacked him. For example, here is Mozart's plaintive request to his father, written when he was 21: "just let me ask you one thing, and that is, not to have such a bad opinion of me. So once more I beg you most humbly to think better of me" (p. 430). In a postscript to this letter, Wolfgang referred to himself in a poem (to his sister and a female friend) as "Mozart, that queerest of fishes" (p. 430). ("Scoundrel" would be a more accurate translation of the phrase [Erna Schwerin, personal communication, November 1990].)

During his old age, Leopold became bitter about his relationship with his son. And Leopold had his reasons for bitterness. He had sacrificed much of his own career for his son's, an occurrence that is common amongst parents of gifted children who may give up their own professional lives for their prodigiously talented children (Feldman, 1986, p. 95).

At his core, Mozart probably felt unloved by egocentric, ambitious Leopold. Mozart was bound to see himself as having failed his father. Mozart received Leopold's adoration and love for what he could do as a musician. But after his childhood Mozart did not receive much love for who he was, nor for what he did, as a person. Leopold's love was conditional. He loved Mozart because of his stupendous talents as a performer on the piano, organ, violin, and viola, and, of course, musical compositions of marvelous diversity.

Leopold's wish to exploit his son's talent can be documented early in Wolfgang's development. When Wolfgang was 11 years old Leopold wrote the following from Vienna to his Salzburg landlord regarding his ambitions for his son:

Or should I perhaps sit down in Salzburg with the empty hope of some better fortune, let Wolfgang grow up, and allow myself and my children to be made fools of until I reach the age which prevents me from travelling and until he attains the age and physical appearance which no longer attract admiration for his merits? Is my child to have taken the first step with this opera for nothing, and is he not to hurry on with firm steps along the road . . . [p. 85].

Leopold tried to influence Wolfgang into a guilty obedience toward him. He often used threats of his own physical disorders in an attempt to bring his headstrong son into line: "As long as I am not anxious about you, I am well" (p. 529); "take care of your health. On yours depends my life . . ." (p. 569). Leopold wanted to remain Wolfgang's closest love object. He wrote to 22-year-old Wolfgang: "There is no true friend . . . but a father" (p. 598).

In his letters to Wolfgang, Leopold's writing style at times resembles that of a forlorn lover. Leopold often indicated that his heart was suffering. Even though Wolfgang and his mother were traveling together, Leopold addressed the following letter "to you [Wolfgang] alone":

> My heart is heavy indeed, now that I know that you will be still farther away from me. . . . you cannot feel the burden of grief which is weighing down my heart. . . . When you were children, I gave up all my time to you in the hope . . . that I might enjoy a comfortable old age. . . . my long life or my speedy death are . . . in your hands" [p. 464].

The important point is that in order for Mozart to earn love from his father, he had to carry out Leopold's wishes. If Mozart wanted to live out his own aspirations, he had to fail his father. This was because Leopold's wishes were so egocentric, unrealistic, and hard to fulfill. But by failing his father, he opened himself to Leopold's condemning criticisms.

Leopold's many criticisms—his "cutting remarks" (Anderson, 1966, p. 172), and statements to the effect that Wolfgang's behavior could "crush" and "kill" (p. 491) him—were an important source of Wolfgang's compromised self-worth.

But Mozart struggled against his father's criticisms. And, as we have seen, he felt justly proud of his gifts as a musician. In fact, the polarities in Mozart's identity and the contradictions in his self-worth may well have helped him to create appealing opera characters with humorous and clownlike characteristics. For example, the bird catcher Papageno in *The Magic Flute* seemed to have had particular meaning for Mozart. Mozart appears to have had a special affection for Papageno, as suggested by the following vignette: "The day before his death, [Mozart] began to hum the bird catcher's song in a scarcely audible voice. Kappellmeister Roser, who was sitting at his bedside, went to the piano and sang the song, to Mozart's evident delight" (Jahns, 1882, vol. 3, p. 356).

Mozart seems to have identified with Papageno. Papageno embodied many of Mozart's own traits. For example, "Simple Simon" (Anderson, 1966, p. 145) and "buffoon" (p. 113) were words Mozart used to describe himself in letters written decades earlier. The same words would describe Papageno well. Mozart used the buffoon or clown aspect of his identity creatively, through his sympathetic and vivid portrayals of buffoonlike personalities in his operas.

We can observe Mozart's sympathetic identification with Papageno through a story recounted by Mozart. The story concerns a scene in which Papageno sings an aria with silver bells (a glockenspiel) in his arms. (Papageno only pretends to play the glockenspiel; the glockenspiel is actually played by another musician from behind the scenes.) During a performance of *The Magic Flute* in Vienna in 1791, 35-year-old Mozart was sitting in the audience in one of the box seats. Here is Mozart's own account of what happened:

> But during Papageno's aria with the glockenspiel I went behind the scenes, as I felt a sort of impulse today to play it myself. Well, just for fun, at the point where Schikaneder [Papageno] has a pause [in his singing], I played an arpeggio. He was startled, looked behind the wings and saw me. When he had his next pause, I played no arpeggio. This time he stopped and refused to go on. I guessed what he was thinking and again played a chord. He then struck the glockenspiel and said "Shut up" [Anderson, 1966, p. 969].

Fortunately, Mozart's prank came off well. Mozart, who loved to clown around, even managed to steal the show by out-clowning the buffoon, Papageno. But why would Mozart suddenly interrupt his music in order to play a boyish prank? By doing so he ran a risk of compromising the performance of his opera. It is difficult to think of another composer of that time engaging in a prank with one of his own operas.

We can discern the workings of two polarities in Mozart's response to the performance of *The Magic Flute*. First we see Mozart as the composer of sublime music, observing the audience—a packed house—enraptured by his music. But it seems that Mozart was not content with this. Mozart experienced a feeling, "a sort of impulse" and could not contain himself any longer. The audacious fool within Mozart simply had to leave the box and join in. Specifically, Papageno's clowning on the stage touched a resonant chord in Mozart—the buffoon chord, the unruly clown, the brilliant audacious "fool" (Anderson, 1966, p. 128) so central to Mozart's identity. Gedo (1986) suggests that "Mozart was asserting that *he* was Papageno," in reference to this passage in Mozart's letters (p. 109).

Why would Mozart act like a buffoon when people were admiring him? Why would he run the risk of playing a prank in his own opera, especially at a time when success was so important to his career? Mozart probably appreciated how much the audience was delighted by his opera and sensed how much they lauded him as a composer. But the public's glorification of him as a composer did not seem to be sufficient to repair his sense of low self-worth.

At many times during his life Mozart must have experienced his father participating vicariously in Mozart's glory. On the other hand, Leopold let Mozart know quite clearly that he did not want Mozart to be a prankster. For example, 21-year-old Mozart wrote his father, "I did . . . perpetrate—rhymes, . . . sheer garbage, that is, on such subjects as muck, shitting and arse-licking—and that too in thoughts, words—but not in deeds. . . . I must admit that I thoroughly enjoyed it. . . . I firmly resolve to go on with the sinful life which I have begun" (Anderson, 1966, p. 373). Leopold replied: "you have just had a holiday and have spent the time in enjoyment and amusement. . . . A journey of this kind is no joke. . . . You should have more important things in your mind than practical jokes; you should be endeavouring to arrange a hundred things in advance, or you will find yourself suddenly in the soup . . ." (pp. 388–389).

Mozart did not heed Leopold's advice. A year later Leopold was still warning Mozart, this time regarding Mozart's relationship with his most important potential supporter in Paris, Baron Friedrich Grimm, German-born secretary to the Duc d'Orleans: "be sure not to play any impudent prank on him," Leopold cautioned him (p. 620). Leopold did not always appreciate his son's personality, a personality which inevitably came along with the wide-ranging musical abilities.

When Mozart played the buffoon, it was as if he were saying to Leopold, and to his audience as well: "You love me for what I could do as a musician, but there are other parts to me—I'm a playful buffoon as well. So there!" In fact, the fool within Mozart would sometimes emerge when he sensed that people were admiring him.

During his adolescence, Mozart portrayed himself as a fool and a buffoon. When Mozart entered adulthood, other people observed that he behaved like a fool and a buffoon. Mozart seemed to be rounding out his expression of who he was, or of who he felt he was, by playing the buffoon. People unconsciously attempt to manipulate and fashion their experiences into events that run true to the images of themselves that are first formed during childhood and adolescence. That is what Mozart did.

In addition to *The Magic Flute*, two of Mozart's other late operas reflect the polarities in Mozart's personality. Mozart wrote that he chose his opera libretti from hundreds of works which he read. In selecting among so many libretti, I assume that he sometimes chose works that struck resonant, dominant chords during particular phases of his psychological development.

Clown characters, or "Hans Wurst" figures as they were called in Vienna (Rosen, 1972, p. 317), appealed to Mozart, perhaps because he was clownlike at times. These characters were "valet buffoons, clowns, and . . . all possessed . . . intelligence . . . and a love of practical jokes . . ." (*Encyclopedia Britannica*, 1974, Micropedia, Vol. 10, p. 863). This description captures some of Mozart's own personality traits. Mozart gave us memorable Hans Wurst figures: Papageno in *The Magic Flute*, Figaro in *The Marriage of Figaro*, and Leporello in *Don Giovanni*. In *The Marriage of Figaro* and *Don Giovanni*, there is dramatic tension between aristocratic men on the one hand, and women of several social classes, valets, servants, and villagers on the other hand. The operas portray conflict between those who have power and those who do not; those who exploit and those who serve; those who win women and those who fail in their attempts.

In *The Marriage of Figaro*, Mozart probed some ambiguities of social status. Almaviva undergoes a transformation in which his power and worth are challenged. Almaviva loses his droit de seigneur, and his hold on women and servants is loosened. As Almaviva descends, the valet Figaro rises in status and power. Not only does Figaro maintain control over his marriage plans, he also discovers that he was born into a higher social class. In *Don Giovanni*, Mozart explored a dark side of male psychology and sexuality. As well, he may have been exploring some dark recesses of his own personality. As Don Giovanni himself loses control over events and spirals downward, he falls to a debased and diabolical status. The shadowy side of Mozart's nature may have been of use to him in creating the powerfully dramatic score of *Don Giovanni*. (By contrast, Beethoven found that the subject matter of *Don Giovanni* was morally unsuitable for opera.)

The two principal noblemen in the two operas, Almaviva and Don Giovanni, descend in status. The valet Figaro rises in his social status. Leporello holds his own at the least, and he experiences an enhancement of his position relative to the fallen status of Don Giovanni. The struggle between the aristocrats and the servants, the elevated and the devalued, creates dramatic power in these operas.

Such a struggle was a relevant one for Mozart. Mozart's father was born into modest circumstances. Leopold's first job was as a "valet and musician" (Turner, 1938, p. 5). The position of "valet" did not, during the eighteenth century, have quite the servile connotation which it does today. Yet Leopold's manner of handling himself with individuals of higher social class was, according to Mozart, "obsequious" (Anderson, 1966, p. 607). Mozart did not want to be like his obsequious father. In view of Mozart's need to separate himself from his father, who died during the writing of *Don Giovanni*, it is striking that, in *Don Giovanni*, a father is murdered just minutes after the curtain rises.

In eighteenth-century Vienna, there existed a huge division of privilege which separated the nobility from the other classes. A court musician, even one such as Mozart, was not considered by the nobility to be a social equal. Mozart dressed like a nobleman, and, when he was not engaging in pranks, he could act like a nobleman. He was relaxed in his dealings with the aristocracy. Yet he was not noble by birth, nor by employment. His ambiguous social position allowed him the advantage of observing aristocrats with the critical eye of an artist. The plots of *The Marriage of Figaro* and *Don Giovanni* question whether valets and other servants should relate to the nobility as they were called upon to do by eighteenth-century conventions. The plots indicate that the nobility are greatly flawed. They were depicted as engaging in egotistical, destructive behavior.

Performance of the Beaumarchais play on which *The Marriage of Figaro* was based had been prohibited in the Austrian Empire by

Emperor Joseph II. The Emperor "instructed his censor that a German translation of *Figaro* should be banned unless expurgated of its more offensive passages" (Heartz, 1990, p. 108) Yet Mozart himself approached a librettist, Da Ponte, to collaborate on the opera. It was a somewhat hazardous project. Singer (1977) stated: "Napoleon cited Beaumarchais's play as one of the major causes of the French Revolution. In its own way, Mozart's opera may have been equally subversive. . . . By striking at the sexual authority . . . [of] the male seducer who also runs the state, Mozart's music relentlessly . . . eats away at the social order, like an ocean endlessly gnawing at the shore" (p. 77).

It appears that the Emperor, who had originally viewed the project of the opera with considerable distaste, "was eventually won over . . . by Mozart playing large parts of the score to him" (Hughes, 1972, p. 49). Count Almaviva's philandering and Figaro's references to women's faithlessness ran the risk of offending the Viennese nobility. "A clever critic . . . pointed up the history of the *Figaro* saga in Vienna in 1785–86 by beginning his review, 'Nowadays what is not allowed to be spoken is sung' " (Heartz, 1990, p. 109). Even though its first performance was well-received, "its popularity was short-lived" (Dent, 1947, p. 97).

Similarly, in *Don Giovanni*, we find Mozart writing an opera which portrays a revolutionary perspective on eighteenth-century social mores. As Rosen (1972) suggested, "an element of liberal revolutionary aspiration is decidedly, if unsystematically, present in [*Don Giovanni*]. No one in 1787 . . . could have missed the significance of Mozart's triumphantly overemphatic setting of 'viva la libertà,' or of the wicked exploitation of peasant innocence for dissolute aristocratic vice" (pp. 322–323).

Fortunately, like Figaro and Leporello, Mozart had a great longing for freedom. Mozart knew all too well the psychology of the relationship of servant to master. The contrast in these two operas between the purportedly high and low ranks of society also existed in Mozart's own elevated and devalued feelings of self-worth. In his own life, Mozart struggled and rebelled against the devalued status of being his father's lifelong servant.

Mozart's self-worth would have been too compromised by remaining in Salzburg and serving his father's needs. In 1781, the 25-year-old Mozart established himself in Vienna. In doing so, he broke away from his father and also from Count Hieronymus Colloredo, the archbishop of Salzburg. By moving to Vienna, Mozart was able to

establish a life for himself that gave him greater psychological freedom and musical scope.

In summary, Mozart made many references about himself which
indicate that he felt compromised in his feelings of self-worth. Mozart's appearance and his father's criticism contributed to his wobbly
self-worth. Even though Mozart was a great genius, he demonstrated
a lack of confidence in his worth as a person. Issues concerning self-
worth can be found among other highly talented individuals. Highly
gifted children and adolescents do not easily get over the trauma of
compromised self-worth. Even for grown-up Wunderkinds, the pains
of adolescence tend to linger on. They may become national figures
in their professions and derive genuine feelings of self-worth from
their achievements, yet they may still bear the scars from childhood
and adolescence. Some of these scars seem to have lingered on in the
personality of one of the great musical geniuses.

What Mozart wrote about himself as an adolescent became true
of him when he was an adult. Significantly, he behaved as an adult in
ways that resembled his "joking" references to himself in adolescence.
He expressed in adulthood the childlike and impulsive, bad boy aspects of himself that were difficult to live out when he was under
Leopold's constricting control.

Mozart also transformed his compromised self-images into fun,
and jests, and art. Mozart's relationship with his father sensitized him
to the issue of exploitation. In his later operas, and elsewhere, Mozart
rebelled by calling into question the eighteenth-century social order
and the hierarchy of noblemen above servants.

What I have described is only part of a complex and rich personality. The buffoon and the fool were part of the man Mozart. We
should not demand of Mozart that he be a genius in all aspects of his
existence.

REFERENCES

Anderson, E. (1966), *The Letters of Mozart and His Family*. New York: W. W.
    Norton, 1985.
Davies, P. (1989), *Mozart in Person*. Westport, CT: Greenwood Press.
Dent, E. (1947), *Mozart's Operas*. Oxford, U.K.: Oxford University Press.
Deutsch, O. E. (1966), *Mozart, A Documentary Biography*. Stanford: Stanford
    University Press.

Encyclopedia Britannica (1974), Zanno. Micropaedia, Vol. 10. Chicago: Encyclopedia Britannica.

Feldman, D. H. (1986), *Nature's Gambit.* New York: Basic Books.

Freud, S. (1905), Jokes and Their Relation to the Unconscious. *Standard Edition,* 8. London: Hogarth Press, 1960.

Gedo, J. E. (1986), Portrait of the artist as adolescent prodigy: Mozart and the magic flute. *Problems of Performing Artists,* September: 107–111.

Heartz, D. (1990), *Mozart's Operas,* ed. T. Baumann. Berkeley: University of California Press.

Hughes, S. (1972), *Famous Mozart Operas.* New York: Dover.

Jahns, O. (1882), *The Life of Mozart,* Vol. 3, trans. P. D. Townsend. London: Novello, Ewer.

Levinger, L. (1979), The intellectually superior child. In: *Basic Handbook of Child Psychiatry,* Vol. 1, ed. J. D. Noshpitz. New York: Basic Books, pp. 328–333.

Marshall, R. (1991), *Mozart Speaks.* New York: Schirmer.

Rosen, C. (1972), *The Classical Style.* New York: W. W. Norton.

Schwerin, E. (1987), *Leopold Mozart, Profile of a Personality.* New York: Friends of Mozart.

Singer, I. (1977), *Mozart and Beethoven.* Baltimore: Johns Hopkins University Press.

Turner, W. J. (1938), *Mozart, the Man and His Works.* New York: Tudor.

6

Mozart and the Vienna World of Medicine: Ideals and Paradoxes

Günter B. Risse, M.D., Ph.D.

HEALTH CONDITIONS

Mozart's birth at Salzburg in January 1756 occurred during a time of intense diplomatic maneuvering by Austria, France, and Russia against Frederick II of Prussia, who had earlier seized Silesia, and deprived the Habsburg monarchy of one of its richest provinces. Coinciding with Mozart's early childhood, the ensuing Seven Years' War pitted the forces of these three powerful European states against an Anglo-Prussian alliance. The period witnessed large scale political intrigue among the allies as well as financial strain for Austria, which was compounded by inept military leadership in the conduct of the war (Gershoy, 1963).

Mozart's status as the seventh—but only the second surviving—child of his parents graphically illustrates the high infant mortality rate affecting all contemporary European countries and social classes (Greither, 1958; Deutsch, 1965; O'Shea, 1990, pp. 25–38). Later, in his own marriage, only two of his six children outlived infancy. The problem was in part nutritional, troubling both mothers and newborns. As one contemporary (Frank, 1790) described it, "sowed in exhausted soil, the fetus has hardly drawn the first juices through the animal roots of the placenta, when, without resistance, it already is shaken and torn as a result of the awful physical labor imposed upon the ill-nourished mother" (p. 93). Multiple and successive pregnancies—Mozart's mother in her early thirties had four such

83

pregnancies in four years—exhausted already debilitated women who were often opposed to breast-feeding. This attitude prompted the transfer of care and feeding of their offspring to wet nurses and servants. Exposure to disease and contaminated water and food supplies were the main cause of the massive loss of infants in Europe (Rosen, 1976; Komlos, 1986; Floud, Wachter, and Gregory, 1990).

Mozart himself was quite aware of these dangers. In a letter written after the birth of his first child in June 1783, he expressed his opposition to wet-nursing although both his mother-in-law and the midwife apparently begged him to procure such services. To make matters worse, many new mothers willing to nurse were suspected of suffering from "milk fever"—probably puerperal fever—a disease believed to be transmitted during breast-feeding. To avoid such additional risks, Mozart and others simply fed the newborn water, a perilous choice. Indeed, Mozart himself (Braunbehrens, 1986) admitted in a letter that "most children here who are brought up on water do not survive" (p. 99). Throughout his life, infant mortality in Vienna remained at about 40 percent.

As in other countries, the key factors affecting nutrition in the Habsburg Empire were insufficient agricultural production, high food prices, and low wages. Malnutrition was endemic. Conditions had apparently been better in the 1740s, causing widespread increases in population, but now, a generation later, more people were competing for limited food supplies. Short and thin, Mozart was part of a veritable eighteenth-century baby boom that affected every corner of Europe. When conscripted into the army, his Austrian cohorts showed signs of stunted physical growth that eventually bottomed out in the 1780s (Komlos, 1989, esp. chapters 2 and 3, pp. 55–165). Mozart's health, in turn, was further compromised by an irregular lifestyle that included the hazards and stresses of eighteenth-century travel.

Moreover, tuberculosis and venereal disease lurked everywhere. A third of the Viennese hospital patients showed signs of pulmonary tuberculosis, categorized as the "morbus Viennensis" (Neuburger, 1921, p. 129). Annually, more than twelve thousand cases of syphilis were also officially reported. While journeying through Europe, Mozart not surprisingly inspected his fellow travelers for signs of disease. "I have too much dread and fear of diseases and too much care for my health to fool around with whores," he told his father at age 25 (Anderson, 1938, Vol. 3, p. 1166). As always, cities were notorious as breeding places for disease. Moving from one place to the next, travelers like the Mozarts were constantly exposed to new ailments for which they lacked adequate immunity. As his father Leopold remarked in 1762, after the young boy had suffered from another eruptive childhood ailment in Vienna: "Wolfgang hat sich naturalisiert"—an equivalent of our concept of "seasoning," meaning he had adapted to Vienna's contemporary spectrum of disease (Levey, 1971; Neumayr, 1988, p. 54).

Another highly visible scourge at this time in Europe was smallpox. Estimates suggest that perhaps as many as 60 million people perished from the disease during the eighteenth century (Hopkins, 1983). Periodic epidemics originating in urban centers such as Vienna quickly spread to an even more vulnerable countryside, as the Mozarts found out in the fall of 1767. Smallpox was not only feared for its considerable mortality rate, but even more for the permanent disfiguration it left on the faces of its victims. When it came calling, mobile upper-class families hastily retreated to their country estates. Although smallpox inoculation measures, designed to create mild cases without scarring, while conferring lifelong protection, were already coming into vogue in other European countries, the Austrian rulers demurred, fearful of accidental contagion and interference in the works of Divine Providence (Langer, 1976). Confronted with the option of inoculating Mozart in 1764 while in Paris, his father Leopold adhered to the prevailing fatalism, leaving the arrival of the disease in his family to "God's mercy" (Neumayr, 1988, p. 56). Three years later, smallpox permanently disfigured Wolfgang's face. Finally, in March 1768, after falling ill herself, Empress Maria Theresa decided to inoculate her remaining family and thereafter the practice became more acceptable in the Habsburg Empire.

Less notorious, but still a potentially devastating threat, was the plague, seemingly contained by a permanent sanitary cordon located at the border with the Ottoman Empire (Lesky, 1957; Bratescu, 1979). Like China's Great Wall, this military barrier extended for over a thousand miles of territory from Croatia on the Adriatic Sea through Serbia, Wallachia, and Transylvania. A chain of lookout posts within musket-shot distance of each other, roving patrols, and a number of quarantine stations and crossing points for goods and persons completed the strict security arrangements. In spite of such elaborate procedures and the constant fumigation of goods, plague sporadically crossed the cordon, although no major outbreaks were reported (Rothenberg, 1973). But by then, plague was gradually retreating from Europe anyway as a result of changes affecting the ecology of the rat, its major carrier.

MEDICAL POLICE

Faced with costly wars abroad and deteriorating living conditions back home, the Austrian rulers realized the futility of seeking revenge for the loss of Silesia. After her alliance against Prussia crumbled, the Empress Maria Theresa sought to end hostilities. The Peace of Paris, signed in 1763 after Mozart celebrated his seventh birthday, inaugurated a welcome twenty-five-year interval of peace between the major European powers. This period of "enlightened despotism" witnessed political and institutional reforms championed by Europe's absolute rulers and aimed at improving economic conditions and the material lot of its inhabitants (Hazard, 1963; Hulme and Jordanova, 1990). In Austria, the rule of Maria Theresa continued until her death in 1780, followed by the reign of her son, Joseph II, between 1780 and 1790. Those peaceful years also closely corresponded with Mozart's life as an active composer and musician.

While part of the reform movement was aimed at curtailing the power of the Church, notably the Jesuits, another series of governmental measures were aimed at breaking down the political and economic barriers to centralized autocratic domination, a difficult and frustrating task in a multiethnic empire such as Austria (Bernard, 1971; Matis, 1981, pp. 189–202; Wangermann, 1981). Among the newly perceived requirements of national power was the need for an expanding population sufficient to improve agricultural production, increase tax collection, and provide for the growing manpower needs of standing national armies. New controls to insure the welfare of Austria's inhabitants included specific policies concerning health-related issues (Risse, 1992). In contemporary mercantilist ideology the term *Policey*, or police, designated a state-sponsored administrative apparatus supervised by a wise ruler, who used such bureaucratic devices to take care of his people. "Medical police," therefore, described programs and institutions responsible for public and personal welfare and hygiene, as well as the regulation of medical education, training, and practice. This constituted a pronatalist, paternalistic, cradle-to-grave approach congenial to absolute rulers who were convinced that they knew what was best for their citizens (Rosen, 1953). At its center, the program of medical police sought to create a coherent health policy that would include everyone, especially the poor and needier segments of society. Not only would such persons receive some form of medical care, but efforts were made to prevent disease through environmental measures designed to improve the public health. Implicit in the new ideology were Lockeian notions of social contract between the state and its people, and Rousseau's ideas about disease and the rise of civilization. The operative goal was to ostensibly "defend" the population against all kinds of social ills, including those which spawned dangerous diseases. The most influential spokesperson for such a program was a German physician, Johann Peter Frank (1745–1821), who in 1777 began publishing his *System einer vollständigen medicinischen Policey* (Lesky, 1975). By 1785, Frank had joined the medical faculty of the University of Pavia and a year later, became the Director General of Public Health for Lombardy, the northern Italian province, then under Austrian control (Lesky, 1973).

To the delight of his despotic masters, Frank to an unprecedented degree recommended a host of regulatory functions that intruded into every aspect of life, from birth through childhood and adolescence, education, choice of marriage and occupation, housing, personal hygienic habits, injuries and diseases, old age, and death. The task was to persuade or force the lower classes to seek and preserve health in exchange for further governmental control of their individual lives. In his presumption that he understood his subjects and knew what was best for them, Joseph II, the "Volkskaiser," adopted many of these views, presented as the rational embodiment of Enlightenment ideals. Perhaps the intent was benevolent, the approach, however, remained arbitrary, heavy-handed, and thus was often counterproductive (Gershoy, 1963, esp. chapters 1–4, 8, pp. 1–106, 197–234; Jordanova, 1980).

A typical example was Joseph II's establishment of a new general hospital in Vienna. With a population of more than a quarter of a million people at the time of Mozart's arrival in 1781, the city had barely over one thousand beds available for the care of the truly sick. In the tradition of Catholic charity going back to the Middle Ages, most of the facilities also functioned as shelters for the homeless and the old, a fact that contributed to high mortality rates and their reputation as gateways to death (Imhof, 1977; Risse, 1986).[1] Indeed, the crowding and mingling probably generated more sickness than the attending physicians in these institutions were capable of curing. But how could this situation be changed? The emperor actually persuaded some inmates to vacate the premises through cash offerings. Street beggars, in turn, were rounded up and transported to the Bavarian frontier where they were unceremoniously dumped across the border. Perhaps, conventional wisdom suggested, less crowded hospitals could now better spend their resources taking care of the sick poor.

As in other spheres of Austrian life, however, questions of efficiency and centralization were constantly raised. Rejecting all contemporary medical advice that small hospitals with one to three hundred beds would be ideal for the proper care and treatment of patients, Joseph II went for the French model of the Hôtel Dieu and proposed a new, centralized, two-thousand-bed medical facility, the *Allgemeines Krankenhaus* (Greenbaum, 1976). Arranged into small twenty-bed wards in a long, two-story building, the new institution accepted its first patients in August 1784. While attempts were made to keep the premises scrupulously clean, hospital diseases such as typhus and puerperal fever contributed to increase institutional mortality to nearly 20 percent, as predicted by the medical experts. Despite frequent royal visits to raise morale, and burdened with a reputation as a house of death, prospective paying patients never materialized, and the Allgemeines Krankenhaus became a medical embarrassment as well as a significant drain on the state's treasury (Lesky, 1967; Bernard, 1975).

MEDICAL REFORMS

In 1749, Gerard van Swieten, personal physician to the Empress, became prominently involved in reforms affecting the University of Vienna, including its medical school. As part of the government's efforts to assume greater power through bureaucratic consolidation, the faculty lost its previous autonomy and the course of studies shortened. With an anatomical theater and establishment of a chemical

---

[1]In my book, I have tried to argue against the "gateways to death" view for the eighteenth-century British hospitals. The Edinburgh Infirmary had a mortality rate of 4 percent.

laboratory and botanical garden, the school began to shed its medieval character. Inspired by Boerhaave's model at Leyden, the university now started offering regular courses in the basic medical sciences of the day (Neuburger, 1921; Lesky and Wandrusza, 1973). By 1753, clinical bedside teaching also became a regular academic subject, to be taught by another student of Boerhaave's, Anton de Haen (1704–1776), at the *Burgerspital* in Vienna (de Haen, 1779, pp. 10–22; Boersma, 1961–1962). Moreover, de Haen received authorization to fill his twelve-bed teaching ward with patients selected from other Viennese hospitals. The same institutions would henceforth also supply cadavers for postmortem examinations and the study of pathological anatomy. An active outpatient department or polyclinic provided an array of ambulatory cases for study (Lesky, 1970; Risse, 1987–1988).

Since the Habsburg rulers were bent on curbing church power, many young men destined for the priesthood shifted careers and became physicians instead. By the 1760s more than three hundred medical practitioners attended patients in Vienna. Meanwhile, to accomplish his multiple academic obligations, de Haen surrounded himself with assistants, one of them Anton Störk (1731–1803), who in the 1760s became famous for his clinical experiments with hemlock in the treatment of cancer at the Bäckenhäusel Hospital (Schweppe, 1982). Another prominent member of the new school was Leopold Auenbrugger (1722–1809), physician-in-chief at the Spanish Hospital who pioneered the immediate percussion of the chest, a method of examination grounded in pathological studies later revised by the French School (Auenbrugger, 1936). Auenbrugger was also a patron of the arts, and both Haydn and Mozart participated in some of his Sunday musical matinees. De Haen's popular replacement in the clinical chair from 1776 to 1787 was Maximilian Stoll (1742–1787), whose promotion of active learning and interest in epidemiology attracted many medical students (Stoll, 1788–1789; Probst, 1968). In 1785, Joseph II created a Medico-Surgical Academy for two-year training courses behind the 1200-bed military hospital. Headed by his *protochirurgus*, Giovanni A. Brambilla (1728–1800), the Imperial Josephinum decisively contributed to improve the knowledge and professional standing of Austrian military surgeons (Brambilla, 1788). Not surprisingly, late eighteenth-century Vienna became one of the most prestigious medical centers in all of Europe (Lesky, 1974, 1981).

DOMESTIC HEALING AND SPA MEDICINE

Time and again Mozart's biographers reported instances of do-it-yourself healing, especially in the hands of his father Leopold. To this day, domestic medicine remains the initial level at which illness is recognized, defined, and treated. Family members, close friends, neighbors, and workmates usually provide the advice and resources (Risse, 1977, pp. 1–8). Just like physicians, eighteenth-century laypersons also argued endlessly about the particular mixture and location of their bodily humors that seemingly determined their physical constitutions and psychological temperaments. Most medical theories stressed the virtues of a moderate life style. For Mozart's perceived hot and sanguine temper, for example, heat producing drinks including wines were seen as especially dangerous.

During that century, prominent physicians wrote a number of health manuals with the aim of educating the laity and dispelling the widespread but pessimistic notion that sickness was an unavoidable evil (Porter, 1985). Although always ready with his own brand of kitchen medicine, Mozart's father subscribed to the prevailing fatalism in matters of life and death. In reference to his son, he wrote that God, who had put this wonder of nature into the world, must also preserve or take him back (Neumayr, 1988). However, given the vagaries of contemporary European travel, it was always prudent to carry some form of first aid kit. By his own admission, Leopold Mozart's medicine bag was well stocked with a strong antacid and cathartic for all kinds of fever: the so-called Margrave powder or *magnesia alba* containing magnesium carbonate, and a *black epileptic powder* with charcoal, valerian, and mother-of-pearl believed to act as a painkiller and antispasmodic (Estes, 1990, pp. 92, 122).

Another important healing option available to Mozart and his contemporaries was the spa. The frequent use of mineral waters for bathing was a tradition stretching back to antiquity (Krizek, 1990; Porter, 1990). By the mideighteenth century, this practice had reached new levels of popularity in central Europe as well as a modicum of medical legitimacy. Indeed, some physicians conducted elaborate chemical analyses of certain waters; others even came to reside nearby, providing explanations as well as elaborate strategies for their use (von Crantz, 1777, pp. 23–28). An early customer was Mozart's mother Anna Maria, who went to Bad Gastein in the summer of 1750, exhausted and upset after three consecutive pregnancies had ended in dead infants.

The story repeated itself in the summer of 1789, when Mozart's wife Constanze, pregnant with their fifth child, was told by her physician to take the water cure at Baden, outside of Vienna. This popular resort located between vineyards at the foot of the Styrian Alps, had been known since Roman times for its warm, sulfurous waters. A number of private residences, lodging houses, and pensions catered mostly to the affluent sick, especially those suffering from skin ailments, gout, and rheumatism (von Crantz, 1777; Hoffmann, 1882). Although Constanze's ostensible reason for seeking the cure was an apparently recurrent varicose ulcer near the ankle, subsequent and expensive visits during the next two summers and the fall of 1791 may have had to do more with a change of scenery and rest than any actual ill. Spa life was always fun and the company exciting. Moreover, the resulting evasion of matrimonial duties, which at this time inevitably ended in successive and exhausting pregnancies, was even more welcome than the smelly waters.

MEDICAL PRACTICE

As today, when sickness became more life-threatening or failed to yield to popular remedies, Mozart and his contemporaries sought the advice of learned physicians. In the case of Maria Theresa, it was her *protomedicus* Gerard van Swieten, who presided over a medical entourage of nearly thirty people that included physicians, surgeons, dentists, apothecaries, and even a surgeon who specialized in hunting accidents. Like most prominent eighteenth-century physicians managing the rich and famous, van Swieten prominently functioned as a life-style director, closely watching Her Majesty's diet and activities. Moreover, as man-midwifery made its debut at midcentury, he also conducted her births with the assistance of a midwife (Lesky, 1973; Wilson, 1985; Schnorrenberg, 1981).

But, how did physicians actually treat their patients? In this regard a perusal of Anton de Haen's hospital practice is quite informative. As already noted, de Haen was responsible for the *clinicum practicum* or practical clinical instruction until his death in 1776. De Haen prided himself on being a true follower of Hippocratic aphorisms, which meant that he closely adhered to the humoral theory of disease.

With the focus on key fluids such as blood, phlegm, bile, and pus, this physician carefully monitored the patient's bodily discharges, paying attention to their perceived physical qualities, including density and acidity. Unlike other colleagues on the Continent, de Haen was therapeutically very conservative, allowing such discharges to occur freely and dispensing only a few herbal preparations if he believed that they could help cool and dissolve those humors that the healing power of nature seemed unable to dislodge from the body. In most fevers, opium and bloodletting were indicated as a form of sedative when the human economy was ostensibly accelerated. Like other Viennese contemporaries, de Haen was seen as a true follower of nature, allowing clinical events to take their chosen course without burdening the sick body with further purgatives and emetics. This strategy was judged either prudent or foolish, depending on the point of view of individual practitioners (de Haen, 1779).

Mozart's own repeated contacts with the Austrian medical profession can only be imperfectly documented. One such early encounter occurred in October 1762, when he fell ill with a fever and rash while performing for the Empress Maria Theresa at the Schönbrunn Palace outside of Vienna. Here Johann A. von Bernhard, a professor of medicine at the local university and later dean of the medical school, was consulted. In 1765, two Dutch physicians treated our musician in the Hague, as he battled with what was said to be a dangerous "nervous" fever requiring opium. Two years later, it was Alexandre L. Laugier, one of the personal physicians attending the Empress, who urged the panicked Mozarts to promptly leave Vienna, given the fact that they were not vaccinated and therefore were vulnerable to the severe outbreak of smallpox in the city. In Salzburg, the family was in the hands of Franz J. Niederl, an official *Provinzialphysikus* attached to the retinue of Mozart's "Arch-oaf" boss, the archbishop, Count Colloredo (Davies, 1989).

During his last years, Mozart was being seen by Sigmund Barisari, a friend and graduate of the local university, also *physicus primarius* at the Allgemeines Krankenhaus who died in 1787. In the tradition of being a life-style manager, Barisari persuaded Mozart to get some exercise through horseback riding. The other was Thomas F. Closset from the same hospital who had also looked after Mozart's wife, Constanze. On occasion, bloodletting was prescribed. In fact, among the musician's posthumous outstanding debts were bills from his bleeder and apothecary. Shortly before Mozart's death, Closset called Dr. Mathias von Sallaba, a senior physician of that same institution, in consultation. Ironically, it was this practitioner who proclaimed that the musician suffered from a "hitziges Frieselfieber," literally a hot fever with rash, which was then believed to be epidemic in the city. The label was transferred to the death certificate. For Constanze, Mozart also sought out Johann Hunczovsky, a professor of surgery at the Josephinum, who recommended using leeches (Hunczovsky, 1783).[2]

In spite of all this doctoring, Mozart, like many of his contemporaries, remained unimpressed with the benefits of Viennese medicine. On March 30, 1787, he signed the book of a friend, a fellow Freemason and language teacher, Johann G. Kronauer, writing: "Patience and tranquility of mind contribute more to cure our distempers than the whole art of medicine" (Landon, 1983, p. 41). This statement is not surprising. In spite of significant advances in understanding the actions of the human machine in health and disease, eighteenth-century medical treatments remained frozen in a time warp that went back more than two thousand years.

Even in death, Mozart became entangled in Josephine burial ordinances that were part of the Emperor's comprehensive medical police or public health program (Braunbehrens, 1986, pp. 99, 413–424).[3] To avoid any cadaveric contamination of the soil and ground water, cemeteries such as St. Mark's, laid out in 1787, were now located outside the city gates. No-frill funeral services in reusable coffins were encouraged with no ceremonies at the gravesite. Interment in linen sacks stacked up in mass graves and covered with unslaked lime became common to accelerate decomposition, thus avoiding contamination, and facilitate early turnover of the gravesites for subsequent interments. In the final analysis, Mozart's was no pauper's burial, but an illustration of practices and ideologies of hygiene imposed by a despotic ruler in the name of rationality and public health (Braunbehrens, 1986).

In conclusion, while European visitors during the late 1700s repeatedly praised the medical preeminence of Vienna and its distinguished practitioners, a contemporary satirical letter focused on the contradictions between medical advances, institutional reforms, and

---

[2]Hunczovsky was a student of Brambilla's who was sent for postgraduate studies to England, France, and Italy. In 1783 he published his medical observations in a book.

[3]Johann P. Frank had already recommended new burial regulations in his work on medical police. Joseph II's ordinances were issued on August 23, 1784.

health: "We have visited the new *Allgemeines Krankenhaus* which is
arranged for those who really get sick. My cousin, however, tells me
that it is actually not that impressive. He says that the true big hospital
is the entire city of Vienna" (Neuburger, 1921).

REFERENCES

Anderson, E., ed. (1938), *W. A. Mozart, The Letters of Mozart and His Family*, 3
 Vols., 4th ed. New York: W. W. Norton, 1989.
Anon. (1787), Bemerkungen über das Civilspital und die Vieharzneischule
 nebst eingestreuten Reflexionen über Mediziner und Medizinanstal-
 ten in Wien. In: *Das alte medizinische Wien in zeitgenössischen Schilder-
 ungen*, ed. M. Neuburger. Wien: M. Perles, pp. 110–111, 1921.
Auenbrugger, L. (1936), On percussion of the chest. *Bull. Inst. Hist. Med.*,
 4:373–403.
Bernard, P. P. (1971), *Jesuits and Jacobins; Enlightenment and Enlightened Despotism in Austria*. Urbana: University of Illinois Press.
——— (1975), The limits of absolutism: Joseph II and the Allgemeines Kran-
 kenhaus. *Eighteenth-Cent. Stud.*, 9:193–215.
Boersma, J. (1961–1962), Antonius de Haen, 1704–1776, life and work. *Ja-
 nus*, 50:264–307.
Brambilla, G. A. (1788), *Discours sur la prééminence et l'utilité de la chirurgie*.
 Bruxelles: E. Flon.
Bratescu, G. (1979), Seuchenschutz und Staatsinteresse im Donauraum
 (1750–1850). *Sudhoffs Arch.*, 63:25–44.
Braunbehrens, V. (1986), *Mozart in Vienna, 1781–1791*. New York: Grove/
 Weidenfeld.
Davies, P. J. (1989), *Mozart in Person: His Character and Health*. Westport, CT:
 Greenwood Press.
de Haen, A. (1779), *Heilingsmethode in dem kaiserlichen Krankenhause zu Wien*,
 trans. E. Platner. Leipzig: Weygand.
Deutsch, O. E. (1965), *Mozart, A Documentary Biography*, trans. E. Bloom, P.
 Branscombe, & J. Noble. Stanford: Stanford University Press.
Estes, J. W. (1990), *Dictionary of Protopharmacology; Therapeutic Practices,
 1700–1850*. Canton, MA: Science History Publ.
Fildes, V. (1986), *Breasts, Bottles, and Babies, A History of Infant Feeding*. Edin-
 burgh: Edinburgh University Press.
Floud, R., Wachter, K., & Gregory, A. (1990), *Height, Health and History;
 Nutritional Status in the United Kingdom, 1750–1980*. Cambridge, U.K.:
 Cambridge University Press.
Frank, J. P. (1790), The people's misery: Mother of diseases. *Bull. Hist. Med.*,
 9:93, 1941.
Gershoy, L. (1963), *From Despotism to Revolution, 1763–1789*. New York:
 Harper Torchbooks.

Greenbaum, L. S. (1976), Health-care and hospital building in eighteenth-century France: Reform proposals of du Pont de Nemours and Condorcet. In: *Studies on Voltaire and Eighteenth Century*, ed. T. Besterman. Oxford: Voltaire Foundation, pp. 895–930.

Greither, A. (1958), *Wolfgang Amade Mozart*. Heidelberg: L. Schneider.

Hazard, P. (1963), *European Thought in the Eighteenth Century*, trans. J. Lewis May. New York: Meridian Books.

Hoffmann, J. (1882), *Der Kurort Baden bei Wien*. Wien: W. Braumüller.

Hopkins, D. R. (1983), *Princes and Peasants, Smallpox in History*. Chicago: University of Chicago Press.

Hulme, P., & Jordanova, L., eds. (1990), *The Enlightenment and Its Shadows*. London, New York: Routledge.

Hunczovsky, J. (1783), *Medicinisch-chirurgische Beobachtungen auf seinen Reisen durch England und Frankreich besonders über Spitäler*. Vienna.

Imhof, A. E. (1977), The hospital in the 18th century: For whom? In: *The Medical Show*, ed. P. Branca. New York: Science History Publ., pp. 141–163.

Jordanova, L. (1980), Medical police and public health: Problems of practice and ideology. *Soc. Social Hist. Med. Bull.*, 27:15–19.

Komlos, J. (1986), Patterns of children's growth in east central Europe in the eighteenth century. *Ann. Hum. Biol.*, 13:33–48.

——— (1989), *Nutrition and Economic Development in the Eighteenth-Century Habsburg Monarchy, An Anthropometric History*. Princeton, NJ: Princeton University Press.

Krizek, V. (1990), *Kulturgeschichte des Heilbades*. Leipzig: Kohlhammer.

Landon, H. C. (1983), *Mozart and the Masons*. New York: Thames & Hudson.

Langer, W. L. (1976), Immunization against smallpox before Jenner. *Scientif. Amer.*, 234:112–117.

Lesky, E. (1957), Die österreichische Pestfront an der k.k. Militärgrenze. *Saeculum*, 8:82–106.

——— (1967), Das Wiener Allgemeine Krankenhaus. Seine Gründung und Wirkung auf deutsche Spitäler. *Clio Medica*, 2:23–37.

——— (1970), The development of bedside teaching at the Vienna Medical School from scholastic times to special clinics. In: *The History of Medical Education*, ed. C. D. O'Malley. Berkeley: University of California Press, pp. 217–234.

——— (1973), Johann Peter Frank and social medicine. *Ann. Cisalpines d'Hist. Sociale*, 4:137–144.

——— ed. (1974), *Wien und die Weltmedizin*. Wien: H. Böhlaus.

——— ed. (1975), *A System of Complete Medical Police; Selections from Johann Peter Frank*. Baltimore: Johns Hopkins University Press.

——— (1981), *Meilensteine der Wiener Medizin*. Wien: W. Maudrich.

——— Wandrusza, A., eds. (1973), Gerard von Swieten. Auftrag und Erfüllung. In: *Gerard van Swieten und seine Zeit*. Wien: H. Böhlaus, pp. 11–33.

Levey, M. (1971), *The Life and Death of Mozart*. New York: Stein & Day.

Matis, H., ed. (1981), *Von der Glückseligkeit des Staates. Staat, Wirtschaft und Gesellschaft in Oesterreich in Zeitalter des aufgeklärten Absolutismus*. Berlin:

Duncker & Humbolt, especially Leuchtenmüller-Bolognese, B. Bevölkerungspolitik zwischen Humanität, Realismus, und Härte.

Neuburger, M. (1921), *Die Wiener medizinische Schule im Vormärz*. Wien: Rikola.

Neumayr, A. (1988), *Musik und Medizin*. Wien: J & V Edition Wien.

O'Shea, J. (1990), *Music and Medicine*. London: Dent & Sons.

Porter, R., ed. (1985), *Patients and Practitioners, Lay Perceptions of Medicine in Pre-Industrial Society*. Cambridge, U.K.: Cambridge University Press.

—— ed. (1990), *The Medical History of Waters and Spas*. London: Wellcome Institute for the History of Medicine.

Probst, C. (1968), Das Krankenexamen: Methodologie der Klinik bei Boerhaave und der ersten Wiener Schule. *Hippokrates*, 39:820–825.

Risse, G. B. (1977), Introduction. In: *Medicine Without Doctors*, ed. G. B. Risse, R. L. Numbers, & J. W. Leavitt. New York: Science History Publ., pp. 1–8.

—— (1986), *Hospital Life in Enlightenment Scotland. Care and Teaching at the Royal Infirmary of Edinburgh*. New York: Cambridge University Press.

—— (1987–1988), Clinical instruction in hospitals: The Boerhaavian tradition in Leyden, Edinburgh, Vienna and Pavia. *Clio Medica*, 21:1–19.

—— (1992), Medicine in the age of enlightenment. In: *History of Medicine in Society*, ed. A. Wear. Cambridge: Cambridge University Press, pp. 149–195.

Rosen, G. (1953), Cameralism and the concept of medical police. *Bull. Hist. Med.*, 27:21–42.

—— (1976), A slaughter of innocents: Aspects of child health in the eighteenth century. *Stud. Eighteenth Cent. Cult.*, 5:293–316.

Rothenberg, G. E. (1973), The Austrian sanitary cordon and the control of the bubonic plague: 1710–1871. *J. Hist. Med.*, 28:15–23.

Schnorrenberg, B. (1981), Is childbirth any place for a woman? The decline of midwifery in eighteenth-century England. *Stud. Eighteenth Cent. Cult.*, 10:398–408.

Schweppe, K. W. (1982), Anton Störck und seine Bedeutung für die Aeltere Wiener Schule. *Med. Hist. J.*, 17:342–356.

Stoll, M. (1788–1789), *Ratio medendi in nosocomio practico Vindobonensi*. Vienna.

von Crantz, H. J. N. (1777), *Gesundbrunnen der oesterreichischen Monarchie*. Wien.

Wangermann, E. (1981), Reform catholicism and political radicalism in the Austrian enlightenment. In: *The Enlightenment in National Context*, ed. R. Porter & M. Teich. Cambridge: Cambridge University Press, pp. 127–140.

Wilson, A. (1985), William Hunter and the varieties of man-midwifery. In: *William Hunter and the Eighteenth Century Medical World*, ed. W. F. Bynum & R. Porter. Cambridge: Cambridge University Press, pp. 343–369.

7

Mozart's Health, Illnesses, and Death

Peter J. Davies, M.D.

The son of a bookbinder in Augsburg, Leopold Mozart (1719–1787) took with distinction the Bachelor of Philosophy degree in 1738 at Salzburg University. A prolific letter writer, Leopold recorded many fine details about the illnesses of his family. His astute powers of observation, combined with his scholarly knowledge of Latin and scientific subjects, made him a gifted amateur physician. In 1747 Leopold married the daughter of the warden of the Foundation of St. Gilgen, Anna Maria Pertl (1720–1778).

Due to the high mortality from infections, the average life expectancy then was only thirty years. Only two of their seven children survived to maturity: the fourth born, a daughter, became known as Nannerl (1751–1829). The seventh born, a son, was Wolfgang Amadeus (1756–1791, the beloved of God), who was destined to give unheard of pleasure to millions with his glorious music.

Mozart's placenta was retained in the womb of his 36-year-old mother, so that manual removal, without an anaesthetic, was performed by the midwife. Fortunately, there were no complications. Wolfgang also survived infantile nourishment with pap, which was the fashion in Salzburg at that time.

Leopold Mozart noted that on October 4, 1762, Wolfgang suffered with catarrh on the mailboat at Linz. This was presumably a streptococcal upper respiratory tract infection rather than a corhyza, since on October 21st the boy was ill with erythema nodosum (Deutsch, 1966, p. 17; Anderson, 1938, Letters 2, 4). Nor in view of subsequent events was tuberculosis a likely cause (Rothman, 1945;

Bett, 1956). Mozart's attending physician Dr. Johann von Bernhard's mistaken diagnosis of "a kind of scarlet fever" led Dr. J. Barraud to postulate that Mozart contracted at this time postscarlatina nephritis, the disease which eventually caused his death from renal failure (Barraud, 1905).

A month later Wolfgang was again ailing while a bystander at a banquet in the Vienna Hofburg. Then, following the homecoming of the Mozart family to Salzburg on January 5, 1763, Wolfgang was immediately ill with fever and rheumatism in his legs, so that he was unable to stand. He recovered after a week or so in bed. This might have been a bout of rheumatic fever (Bär, 1972, p. 94), but there are insufficient details to be sure. John O'Shea has proposed that it might have been an early manifestation of poststreptococcal Schönlein-Henoch syndrome (O'Shea, 1990, p. 29).

And so already there is evidence in Mozart of a peculiar vulnerability to develop immune complex disease after streptococcal infection. Such susceptibility, possibly aggravated by a chronic septic focus in his tonsils, is likely to have caused his premature death, as we will see.

While the four tours between 1762 and 1771, which occupied seven years of Mozart's life, no doubt contributed to the early maturation of his musical genius, they also exposed him to the many endemic and epidemic diseases of those times. Travelers were especially at risk of contracting endemic diseases, since they often lacked the immunity of the local population.

Though a corhyza at Coblenz during the early fall of 1763 was of minor concern, Wolfgang was in danger of choking during a nasty bout of quinsy in Paris in February 1764, while composing his *Violin Sonatas* (K. 7, 8, 9). He suffered further bouts of upper respiratory tract infection three months later in London, and in Lille the following August.

During the fall of 1765 in the Hague, first Nannerl and then Wolfgang contracted a serious bout of typhoid fever which brought them close to death's door (Shapiro, 1968). Throughout both illnesses the Mozart parents alternated six-hour shifts at their sick child's bedside. They found strength in prayer and arranged for special masses to be offered. The clinical details noted by Leopold in his letters of November 5 and December 12 to Lorenz Hagenauer are a unique reflection of his remarkable perception (Anderson, 1938, Letters 39, 40). Following its onset on November 15, Wolfgang had recovered sufficiently to give a concert on January 22nd. While convalescing at the Hague from typhoid fever, Mozart composed his *Symphony in B-flat* (K. 22).

Soon after arriving in Munich in November 1766, Wolfgang was ill for twelve days with a second febrile bout of rheumatism, so that he could not stand on his feet or move his toes or knees (Anderson, 1938, Letters 45, 46).

On October 26, 1767, Wolfgang came down with smallpox which he had contracted during an epidemic in Vienna. His eyes were inflamed so that Dr. Joseph Wolff forbade him to read or write for several weeks (Anderson, 1938, Letters 52, 53). Nannerl, who also caught it, noted that her brother's face was permanently disfigured by the scars of smallpox.

In 1819 Nannerl informed Joseph Sonnleithner that soon after his return from Italy her 16-year-old brother suffered a serious illness, which was reflected in a portrait of him looking sickly and very yellow. Otto Deutsch concluded this might have been the miniature on ivory attributed to Martin Knoller in Milan in 1773 (Deutsch, 1966, pp. 520–521). Aloys Greither proposed that this illness might have been an acute poststreptococcal nephritis (Greither, 1967), but there are no symptoms or special features to support this diagnosis. Surely Nannerl's description strongly implies the presence of jaundice, so that viral hepatitis (Davies, 1989, pp. 47–48) or less likely, yellow fever (Shapiro, 1968, p. 19) would appear more credible.

Mozart's mother died in Paris on July 3, 1778, aged 57. Her fatal illness, lasting seventeen days, commenced with diarrhea and headache, then progressed with shivers, fever, deafness, hoarseness, delirium, and coma. The likely diagnosis is louse-borne typhus fever (Davies, 1989, pp. 48–49).

Mozart married Constanze Weber (1762–1842) in St. Stephen's Cathedral, Vienna on August 4, 1782. The following May he was stricken with a respiratory tract infection which was prevalent in Vienna at the time. A blood-letting was performed by his friend Dr. Franz Wenzel Gilowsky, the best man at his wedding. His symptoms of severe sore throat, headache, and stabbing pains in the chest suggested tonsillitis and pleurisy. In the letter of June 7, 1783, to his father, Wolfgang made light of this illness which "left me a cold as a remembrance" (Anderson, 1938, Letter 491).

Only two of Mozart's six children survived to maturity—Carl Thomas Mozart (1784–1858) and Franz Xaver Wolfgang Mozart

(1791–1844). The younger son shared the same rare left external ear malformation as his illustrious father—the so-called Mozart Ear—which is inherited as an autosomal dominant trait.

The well-known concurrent association between certain ear malformations and congenital anomalies of the renal tract led two authors to propose that Mozart suffered a renal anomaly such as polycystic kidneys, which caused his death from uremia (Karhausen, 1987), or even from a subarachnoid hemorrhage from a burst Berry aneurysm (Rappoport, 1986). However, a detailed review of the literature on Mozart Ear reveals that it is a benign, isolated defect without any documented association with polycystic kidneys or serious renal tract anomaly. Furthermore an autopsy established that Franz Xaver Wolfgang Mozart died of gastric cancer (Davies, 1987).

Mozart's serious illness during the late summer of 1784 offers an important clue as to the cause of his premature death. Unfortunately Wolfgang's letter to his father with the details is missing, but Leopold relayed the information to Nannerl in a letter dated September 14 (Anderson, 1938, Letter 518). Along with several other people in Vienna at the time, Mozart contracted a "septic rheumatic fever" which afflicted him for six weeks. Treated by his childhood friend, Dr. Sigmund Barisari (1758–1787), the symptoms included fever, chills, drenching sweats, multiple joint pains, and recurrent abdominal colic associated with violent vomiting. No other details are known. Such a history is consistent with rheumatic fever (Bär, 1972, p. 121) or a poststreptococcal Schönlein-Henoch Syndrome with the insidious onset of glomerulonephritis (Davies, 1989, pp. 53–56). During his convalescence from this illness, Mozart completed his *Piano Concerto in B Flat* (K. 456), the *Piano Sonata in C Minor* (K. 457), and the *String Quartet in B Flat* (K. 458).

During the spring of 1787 Leopold Mozart suffered with heart failure. He died suddenly on May 28, aged 67 years, and he was buried that same day.

Between April and August 1790 Mozart was unwell with a variety of physical and mental symptoms. He was wearing head bandages for headache and was also troubled with rheumatic pains, toothache, malaise, fever, chills, and insomnia from pain. Mozart was ill and consumed by worries and anxieties. Little wonder that in 1790 he completed only eight compositions, though they included four masterpieces.

These symptoms were recounted in his letters to his fellow Free-mason, Michael Puchberg (1741–1822), interspersed with pitiful, desperate pleas for loans to pay off his debts (Anderson, 1938, Letters 576, 578, 583). New light has been shed on these debts by the recent discovery that Mozart was successfully sued for 1460 gulden in November 1791, just six weeks before his death, by Prince Carl Lichnowsky (1756–1814), who had taken him to Leipzig in 1789 (Brauneis, 1991). Presumably this was a gambling debt settled anonymously by the Masons, as there was no mention of it in the inventory of Mozart's estate.

While the above symptoms, taken in isolation, are too vague to permit an accurate diagnosis, the recent research on the skull in the Mozarteum might shed new light on the problem. It is alleged that at the time of Mozart's burial in a group grave (Schachtgräber), the sexton of St. Mark's cemetary, Joseph Rothmayer, identified his corpse, so that when the grave was reopened in 1801 for further use, he pilfered Mozart's skull. It passed on in turn to his successor, Johann Joseph Radschopf, then it passed to the musician and copper engraver, Jacob Hyrtl, and finally to his brother, the eminent Viennese anatomist and anthropologist, Professor Joseph Hyrtl (1810–1894), who made a detailed study of it (*Wiener Fremdenblatt*, 1875; Davies, 1989, pp. 171–174).

The recent research of Puech, Tichy, and coworkers has concluded that the skull is probably genuine. A positive identification with Mozart was established by the techniques of study of the craniofacial indices, portrait superimposition, and dental aging. This is the skull of a young male ultrabrachycephalic central European caucasian, aged between 25 and 40 years (Puech, Puech, and Tichy, 1989; Tichy, 1989). The fascinating pathological findings in this skull include a consolidated fracture in the left temperoparietal region, associated with a chronic, calcified extradural hematoma, and also dental caries, which is most marked in the first left upper molar, with lesser decay in the second (Puech, Puech, Dhellemmes, Pellerin, Lepoutre, and Tichy, 1989, 1990).

However, the Mozarteum in Salzburg commissioned further independent studies by Viennese anthropologists and forensic specialists. There was controversy about the nature of the anomaly of the metopic suture (Bahn, 1991). Then in May 1991 the Mozarteum issued an official statement that, according to the status of current research on the skull in its possession, scientific proof was lacking that the skull was that of Mozart.

It therefore seems likely that Mozart's headache and toothache in 1790 were due to a dental abscess, rather than an extradural hematoma following a head injury. His rheumatic pains may have been related to immune complex disease, while there may have also been an exacerbation of his cyclothymic depression (Davies, 1989, pp. 58–59, 156–157).

During the latter half of 1791 Mozart showed evidence of chronic ill health. While composing *Die Zauberflöte* and the *Requiem* he was subject to strange fainting fits with loss of consciousness for several minutes (Rochlitz, 1798, pp. 147–149, 177–178; Jahn, 1882, III, p. 353). During his visit to Prague for the production of *La Clemenza di Tito*, Mozart became ill and was continually receiving medical attention (*Krönungs Journal für Prag*, 1791, pp. 382–384). His friend Niemetschek noted that his complexion was pale and that his melancholic mood was sometimes interspersed with merry jesting in the company of his friends. Soon after his return to Vienna in the middle of September Mozart informed his wife in the Prater that he was composing the *Requiem* for himself, and then, with tears in his eyes, he continued, "I feel definitely that I will not last much longer; I am sure I have been poisoned. I cannot rid myself of this idea" (Niemetschek, 1956, p. 43).

Such paranoid delusions, in association with probable anemia, and also a history of loin pain and weight loss are compatible with uremic cerebral vascular disease (Barraud, 1905, p. 744; Slater and Meyer, 1960; Greither, 1967, p. 725; Davies, 1989, pp. 61–65).

Mozart's fatal illness commenced on November 20, 1791, and lasted fifteen days. It was precipitated by an infection contracted in an epidemic. Dr. Guldener von Lobes (1763–1827) stated that several other inhabitants of Vienna at that time died with similar symptoms (Deutsch, 1966, p. 523).

Nissen informed us that Mozart was confined to bed during this illness which "commenced with swelling of the hands and feet and an almost complete immobility: after which followed sudden vomiting. . . . Until two hours before he passed away he remained in full possession of his senses" (Nissen, 1984, p. 572).

This account in Nissen, obtained from his wife, together with the eyewitness statements of Sophie Haibel (1763–1846), Joseph Eybler (1765–1845), and Benedict Schack (1758–1826), along with the only two medical documents, constitute the original sources. The controversial issues are the interpretation of his swollen condition and almost complete immobility, together with the question of a rash.

The evidence in favor of a polyarthritis is threefold. Sophie Haibel informed the Novellos that Mozart's arms and limbs were much inflamed and swollen (Medici and Hughes, 1955, p. 215). Eybler stated that "in his painful final illness I helped to lift him up, lay him down, and wait upon him" (1826, p. 338; see also Maunder, 1989, p. 14). Furthermore, Dr. Guldener's diagnosis of a rheumatic inflammatory fever (una febbre reumatico inflammatoria) leaves no doubt that there was an inflammatory affliction of Mozart's joints (Deutsch, 1966, p. 522; Bär, 1972, p. 57).

However, it would appear that in addition there was also a generalized edema, due to fluid retention, which progressed to an anasarca. In an undated note, discovered amongst the personal effects of Carl Thomas Mozart, it was stated that the gross swelling of Mozart's corpse rendered an autopsy impossible (Dalchow, Duda, and Kerner, 1971, p. 231). While the latter conclusion is nonsense, the note does highlight the marked degree of edema.

Yet the combination of polyarthritis and generalized edema should not have caused an almost complete immobility. Sophie Haibel informed Nissen that she and her mother made a night-jacket for Mozart which could be put on from the front, since on account of his swollen condition he was unable to turn over in bed by himself (Anderson, 1938, p. 975). Schack stated that "his weakness was such, that he was obliged to be drawn forward whenever he required to sit up in bed" (*Allgemeine Musikalische Zeitung*, 1827, pp. 519–521; see also Holmes, 1845, p. 347). Eybler informed us that Mozart had to be lifted into and out of bed. Holmes translated the relevant passage in Nissen ("Einer beynahe gänzlichen Unbeweglichkeit") as "an almost total incapacity of motion" (Holmes, 1845, p. 346). Jahn expressed it slightly differently, which in translation became: "partial paralysis set in" (1882, pp. 111, 354; Davies, 1991). The weakness is best accounted for by a muscular paralysis which was most likely to have been a hemiplegia.

Since October 1791 or earlier, Mozart was attended by Dr. Thomas Franz Closset (1754–1813), who had witnessed the evolution of neuropsychiatric symptoms. Closset suspected that Mozart was suffering from a serious intracranial lesion for he diagnosed "un deposito alla testa," literally a deposit in the head. However, Closset was puzzled by the onset of a febrile illness associated with painful swollen joints, gross edema, and an almost complete immobility.

On November 28 Closset called in consultation Dr. Mathias von Sallaba (1754–1797) who diagnosed "Hitziges Frieselfieber," a high miliary fever, the entry in the Register of Deaths. A rash must therefore have been present since the term *Miliaria* ("Friesel" in German) was derived from an eruption of distinct papules or vesicles, of the size of millet seeds, pinheads, or hemp seeds (Hebra, 1866–1880, I, p. 383; Davies, 1991). In his treatise on *Der Friesel*, Franz Seitz outlined the diverse clinical spectrum which contrasted a sporadic exanthemlike purpura at one end, extending through a contagious disease, even occurring in endemic or epidemic forms, at the other (Seitz, 1852; Davies, 1991).

On the last night, at about 11 o'clock, following the application of a cool towel to his forehead, Mozart convulsed and became unconscious. Toward midnight he attempted to raise himself, opened his eyes, and then fell back with his face turned to the wall. His cheek was puffed out and he died an hour later (Anderson, 1938, p. 977). These symptoms, suggestive of paralysis of conjugate gaze and facial nerve palsy, are compatible with massive hemorrhage in either one of the frontal lobes or brain stem.

The cause of Mozart's death has been discussed in detail elsewhere (Davies, 1989, pp. 195–205). The absence of a history of breathlessness is strong evidence against a diagnosis of rheumatic fever causing heart failure. Nor does rheumatic fever account well for the immobility or cerebral hemorrhage. While in the absence of an autopsy we will never be certain as to the cause of Mozart's death, all the symptoms of his fatal illness, contracted during an epidemic, are well accounted for only by the diagnosis of Schönlein-Henoch Syndrome, which is also favored by other scholars (Green and Green, 1987; O'Shea, 1990, p. 35). Furthermore, the Schönlein-Henoch Syndrome diagnosis is in keeping with Mozart's peculiar vulnerability to develop immune complex disease following streptococcal infection.

Mozart's gross edema is also well accounted for by the Schönlein-Henoch Syndrome, where three mechanisms may be responsible. First, there may be localized angioedema, even in the absence of renal involvement. Second, in glomerulonephritis fluid retention may be related to an acute nephritic syndrome, a nephrotic syndrome, or renal failure. Third, edema may be aggravated by hypoproteinemia from a protein-losing gastroenteropathy.

Soon after Mozart's death, Count Joseph Deym, alias Müller (1752–1804), came to take a plaster cast of the composer's face. Subsequently, a wax figure of Mozart dressed in his own clothing was exhibited at Müller's art gallery. Following the death of Deym and his widow, the gallery was liquidated and Mozart's death mask vanished. There is controversy over the authenticity of the bronze death mask now owned by Dr. Gunther Duda (1985; Davies, 1989, pp. 174–177).

The ridiculous allegations that Mozart was poisoned have been detailed elsewhere (Davies, 1989, pp. 179–194). Such allegations took their origin not only in the mental delusions of Mozart and Antonio Salieri (1750–1825), but also in the common knowledge that heavy metal poisoning may give rise to gross dropsy.

The poisoning hypotheses are inconsistent with the epidemic nature of Mozart's fatal illness. Dr. Guldener von Lobes specifically stated that "the very slightest suspicion of his having been poisoned entered no one's mind" (Deutsch, 1966, p. 523).

It will suffice to add that the more specific features of poisoning with aqua toffana or corrosive sublimate were absent in Mozart. The major toxic ingredients of aqua toffana are the oxides of arsenic, lead, and antimony. However, there was absence in Mozart of a blue gum line, peripheral neuropathy, and the characteristic dermatitis. Likewise, there was an absence of such characteristic features of mercury poisoning as tremor, speech disturbance, salivation, chronic gingivitis, and erythism.

There is much interest in the recent discovery that Emanuel Schikaneder (1751–1812) conducted the Vienna court orchestra in a performance of Mozart's *Requiem*, shortly after the composer's death, at a hitherto unknown memorial service in St. Michael's Church in Vienna (Robbins Landon and Robbins Landon, 1991). The absence of tremor in Mozart's hand in the last page of the autograph of the *Requiem*, and in the last entries of his personal thematic *catalogue*, is convincing evidence that he was not poisoned with mercury. Let the fantastic myths that Mozart was poisoned be laid to rest forever.

REFERENCES

Allgemeine Musikalische Zeitung (1827), A posthumous tribute to Benedict Schack. July 25:519–521.
Anderson, E. (1938), *The Letters of Mozart and His Family*, 3rd ed. London: Macmillan, 1985.

Bahn, P. G. (1991), The face of Mozart. *Archaeology*, 44:38–41.
Bär, C. (1972), *Mozart: Krankheit. Tod. Begräbnis*, 2nd ed. Salzburg, Austria: Int. Stift. Mozarteum.
Barraud, J. (1905), A quelle maladie à succombe Mozart? *La Chronique Médicale*, 12:737–744.
Brauneis, W. (1991), Owing to indebtedness of 1,435 Gulden 32 Kreuzer: A new document on Mozart's financial plight in November 1791, trans. B. C. Clark. *Mitteilungen der Internationalen Stiftung Mozarteum, Salzburg*, 39:159–163.
Bett, W. R. (1956), W. A. Mozart: A puzzling case-history. *Med. Press*, 90.
Dalchow, J., Duda, G., & Kerner, D. (1971), *Mozarts Tod (1791–1971)*. Pähl, Germany: Verlag Hohe Warte.
Davies, P. J. (1987), Mozart's left ear, nephropathy and death. *Med. J. Australia*, 147:581–586.
―――― (1989), *Mozart in Person: His Character and Health*. Westport, CT: Greenwood Press.
―――― (1991), Mozart's death: A rebuttal of Karhausen: Further evidence for Schönlein-Henoch Syndrome. *J. Roy. Soc. Med.*, 84:737–740.
Deutsch, O. E. (1966), *A Documentary Biography*, 2nd ed., trans. E. Blom, P. Branscombe, & J. Noble. London: Adam & Charles Black.
Duda, G. (1985), *Der Echtheitsstreit um Mozarts Totenmaske*. Pähl, Germany: Verlag Hohe Warte.
Eybler, J. (1826), Selbstbiographie. *Allgemeine Musikalische Zeitung* (Leipzig). May 24:338.
Green, S. T., & Green, F. A. M. (1987), The great composers: Their premature deaths. *J. Roy. Coll. Physicians*, 21:202–205.
Greither, A. (1967), Die Todeskrankheit Mozarts. *Deutsch. Med. Wschr.*, 92:723–726.
Hebra, F. (1866–1880), *On Diseases of the Skin Including the Exanthemata*, 5 vols., trans. C. Hilton Fagge. London: New Syndenham Society.
Holmes, E. (1845), *The Life of Mozart*. London: Chapman & Hall.
Jahn, O. (1882), *Life of Mozart*, 3 vols, trans. P. D. Townsend. London: Novello, Ewer.
Karhausen, L. (1987), Mozart's ear and Mozart's death. Letter. *Brit. Med. J.*, 294:511–512.
Krönungsjournal für Prag (1791), Prague: Albrecht.
Maunder, R. (1989), *Mozart's Requiem: On Preparing a New Edition*. Oxford: Clarendon Press.
Medici, N., & Hughes, R. (1955), *A Mozart Pilgrimage*. London: Novello.
Niemetschek, F. (1956), *Life of Mozart*, trans. H. Mautner. London: Leonard Hyman.
Nissen, G. N. von (1984), *Biographie W. A. Mozarts*. Hildesheim: Georg Olms Verlag.
O'Shea, J. (1990), *Music and Medicine: Medical Profiles of Great Composers*. London: J. M. Dent.
Puech, B., Puech, P-F., Dhellemmes, P., Pellerin, Ph., Lepoutre, F., & Tichy, G. (1989), Did Mozart have a chronic extradural haematoma? *Injury*, 20:327–330.

———— ———— ———— ———— ———— ———— (1990), W. A. Mozart: Craniofacial anaomalies and pathology. *Anthropologie*, 28:67–78.

Puech, P-F., Puech, B., & Tichy, G. (1989), Identification of the cranium of W. A. Mozart. *Forensic Sci. Internat.*, 41:101–110.

Rappoport, A. E. (1986), Mozart's primary disease and cause of death: A multiple congenital malformation syndrome based on a genetic, clinical and pathological study. *Abstr. XVI Int. Congr. Acad. Pathol.*, G, 476.

Robbins Landon, H. C., & Robbins Landon, E. (1991), Wintering in Salzburg. *Musical Times*, 132:203–204.

Rochlitz, F. (1798), Verbürgte Anekdoten aus Wolfgang Gottlieb Mozarts Leben. *Allgemeine Musikalische Zeitung* (Leipzig), 147–149; 177–178.

Rothman, S. (1945), Erythema Nodosum in the 18th century: The case of the child Mozart. *Arch. Dermatol. & Syphilol.*, 52:33.

Shapiro, S. L. (1968), Medical history of W. A. Mozart. *Eye, Ear, Nose & Throat Monthly*, 47:17–20.

Seitz, F. (1852), *Der Friesel, eine historisch.—patholog. Untersuchung.* Erlangen: Verlag von F. Enke.

Slater, E., & Meyer, A. (1960), Contributions to a pathography of the musicians: 2. Organic and psychotic disorders. *Confinia Psychiatrica*, 3:130–131.

Tichy, G. (1989), Zur Anthropologie des Genies: Mozarts Schädel. *Jahrbuch der Universitat Salzburg 1985–1987.* Salzburg: University of Salzburg.

Wiener Fremdenblatt (1875), Mozarts Schädel. October 24.

8

Mozart: Composer and Performer

Paul Hersh

Mozart's documented history as a performer began in his fourth year. In a music book he shared with his talented sister Nannerl, his father wrote beneath a Scherzo by Wagenseil, "This piece was learned by Wolfgangerl on 24 January 1761, three days before his fifth birthday, between nine and nine-thirty in the evening." Less than one year later, on January 12, 1762, Leopold and his two children left for a three-week visit to Munich where both children appeared privately before the Bavarian Elector, Maximilian the Third.

Mozart's first public appearance was at the Trinity Inn in Linz on October 1, 1762. It is interesting that performance during this time consisted not only of playing a piece of music but of improvisation, of playing on different instruments, and in Mozart's case, of singing and playing the violin as well. The touring schedule in the first few years of Mozart's life is truly remarkable. For instance, in 1763 when Mozart was 7, the family left Salzburg on June 9 and began a tour around Europe that lasted three-and-a-half years. Documentary evidence of Mozart's early performances is quite enlightening to study, especially when one reads between the lines.

On the first of December 1763, Friedrich Melchior Von Grimm, a diplomat and man of letters, wrote as follows:

[Mozart], who will be seven years old next February, is such an extraordinary phenomenon that one is hard put to believe what one sees with one's eyes and hears with one's ears. It means little for this child to perform with the greatest precision the most difficult pieces, with hands that can hardly stretch a sixth; but what is really incredible is to see him improvise for an hour on end and in doing so give rein to the inspiration of his genius and to a mass of enchanting ideas, which moreover he knows how to connect with taste and without confusion. . . . The most consummate Kapellmeister could not be more profound than he in the science of harmony and of modulations, which he knows how to conduct by the least expected but always accurate paths. He has such great familiarity with the keyboard that when it is hidden from him by a cloth spread over it, he plays on this cloth with the same speed and with the same precision. To read at sight whatever is submitted to him is child's play for him; he writes and composes with marvelous facility, without having any need to go to the harpsichord and grope for his chords. I wrote him a minuet with my own hand and asked him to put a bass to it; the child took a pen and, without approaching the harpsichord, fitted the bass to my minuet . . . here is something more I have seen, which is no less incomprehensible. A woman asked him the other day whether he was able to accompany by ear, and without looking at it, an Italian cavatina she knew by heart; and she began to sing. The child tried a bass that was not absolutely correct, because it is impossible to prepare in advance the accompaniment to a song one does not know; but when the tune was finished, he asked her to begin again, and at this repeat he not only played the whole melody of the song with the right hand, but with the other hand added the bass without hesitation; whereafter he asked ten times to begin again, and at each repeat he changed the style of his accompaniment; and he could have repeated this twenty times, if he had not been stopped. I cannot be sure that this child will not turn my head if I go on hearing him often; he makes me realize that it is difficult to guard against madness on seeing prodigies. I am no longer surprised that Saint Paul should have lost his head after his strange vision . . . [Deutsch, 1965, p. 26].

It was thought that Mozart did not truly improvise but that he somehow worked the music out in advance. Proof to the contrary was offered when someone gave him a theme that he had never seen before and he did the same thing. Mozart's inventiveness is, I think, the feature that is most remarkable here, not simply his dexterity, but his ability on the occasion to conjure and to find new material and ideas of such wealth and abundance.

From the *Avant-Courier*, a Paris newspaper, on March 5, 1764, we have this report:

[Herr Mozart's] son, who this month reached his eighth year, is a veritable prodigy. He has all the talent and all the science of a maître de chapelle. He plays from memory for hours and, giving rein to the inspiration of his genius, he joins the most valuable ideas to the most profound science of harmony . . . [Deutsch, 1965, p. 30].

A delightful anonymous poem about the Mozart children was given to their father that same month:

Mortals belov'd of God and Kings,
What pow'r doth harmony possess!
When modulated sounds your playing brings,
What taste, what science do you not profess!
Science alone can serve to praise you best.
With what emotion doth wood vibrate!
With sound and sense dumb things you can invest.
Nothing's impossible to you, O mortals blest,
For touch itself with grace you animate [Deutsch, 1965, p. 31].

Part of that three-and-a-half-year trip was spent in England, where an advance notice of the Mozart children's concerts appeared, which read in part:

Taking the opportunity of representing to the Public the greatest Prodigy that Europe or Human Nature has to boast of. Every Body will be astonished to hear a child of such tender Age playing the Harpsichord in such a Perfection—It surmounts all Fantastic and Imagination, and it is hard to express which is more astonishing, his Execution upon the Harpsichord playing at Sight, or his own Composition . . . [p. 34].

And there was one week in London where the children were on display every day for three hours at a local hall. Part of the game at these daily concerts was that you could set challenges; raise the net and Mozart, a boy of only 8, would jump over it.

In Paris the following year, Mozart revealed himself as a singer and organist. In a report from Grimm's *Correspondance Literaire* (originally in French):

[A]lthough his voice is excessively weak, he sings with as much taste as soul. But what is most baffling of all is the profound knowledge of harmony and its most recondite progressions which he possesses to a supreme degree, and which caused the Hereditary Prince of Brunswick, a very competent judge in this matter to say that many Kapellmeisters who have reached the summit of their art will die without ever knowing what this child of nine knows.

Gabriel Cramer (Voltaire's publisher) wrote of Mozart in Geneva in September 1766:

We have here a young German who is strongly recommended to me from Paris, nine years of age; he plays the harpsichord as it has never been played; he reads everything at sight in a moment; he composes instantly on every possible theme; with all that he is gay, child-like, high-spirited, in short one dare not describe him for fear of not being believed [Deutsch, 1965, p. 59].

From Lausanne, October 1766:

You will have seen, with as much surprise as pleasure, a child of nine play the harpsichord like the great masters; & what will astonish you even more was to hear from trustworthy persons that he already played it in a superior manner three years ago; to know that almost everything he plays is of his own composition; to have found in all his pieces, and even in his improvisations, that force of character which is the stamp of genius, that variety which proclaims the fire of imagination & that charm which proves an assured taste . . . [p. 61].

From the periodical *Aristide ou Le Citoyen* appeared this review:

When I see young Mozart jokingly create these tender and sublime symphonies which one would take for the language of immortals, every fibre of my being takes up the theme, so to speak, of immortality, just as all the powers of my spirit despair of it. Carried away by a delightful illusion, beyond the narrowest sphere which confines my senses, I could almost take this child, so blest by heaven, for one of those pure spirits who inhabit the happy realm destined for me [p. 66].

It is important to get beyond the virtuosity and to grasp the fact that all these reports stress something of the soul, of the expression of the depth of feeling in the music as well. I want to give just a couple examples of what I think makes Mozart's music truly great: These illustrations are from the *Piano Sonata in B Flat*, K. 333.

Example 8.1 is just the few opening measures of the first movement:

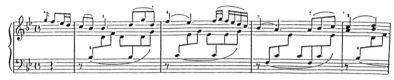

Example 8.1

We need our ears cleaned out, because it is easy to hear this as a bright and overt composition *only*. I am going to rewrite it (Example 8.2):

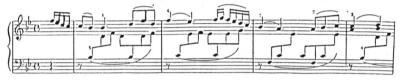

Example 8.2

What I have done is essentially to change one note; but leaving out that one note and the consequent harmony that it leads to changes the entire meaning of the music. Because Mozart starts this sonata, in the key of B flat, on a G. With our jaded ears it is hard to notice that G is the note on which this piece begins. When you hear the spanning interval you see the way Mozart picks that up in the very end of the measure and turns to a world of dark shadow in the minor harmony one measure later. Then, taking the implications of this interval and returning to it, he opens the door to the dominant chord which provides a resolution. When I leave that out and I do what a more ordinary composer might have done, suddenly the whole piece, like a soufflé that has been kept too long, falls flat. The wealth of experience simply is not there.

Now if I return to my poor version (Example 8.3):

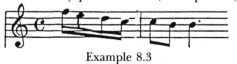

Example 8.3

and I continue with the sequel, it has no meaning because you haven't had the other experience, the moment of darkness and of crisis. The easy route out doesn't work: Before you arrive at paradise, you must go through hell and purgatory. This little pain and its resolution suggest both what is wonderful and difficult in performing Mozart's music. It is critical to express this element, and yet it must be of the utmost, unaffected simplicity and naturalness. In other words, the notes have implications that go deeper than a one-sided interpretation of them.

Two more examples to illustrate how these notes have implications far deeper than a one-sided interpretation of them. The outline of the opening configuration stripped bare is this (Example 8.4):

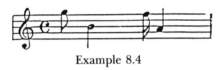

Example 8.4

Mozart introduces those outer parametric bounds and then picks up that exact figure in the concluding passage in a way that reveals its simplest cadential meaning (Example 8.5):

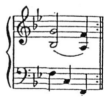

Example 8.5

But in the harmonic developmental sequence relating to this simple outline (measure 44), if you change the bass and take away Mozart's absolutely inspired C sharp (example 6A), all you get is something quite pleasant. It would just have been so easy to let the pen fall and conclude in the way it began, and yet, to paraphrase Wordsworth, "oh, the difference the difference it makes." It is truly amazing. That C sharp pushes up in the bass and you feel a different emotion touched, something you hardly expected at that moment, yet so revealing in its unexpectedness, especially if you put it in its context.

This is what makes Mozart's music absolutely amazing: the setting up of a context so that there can be these variations of experience, these little touches that are so deep and profound and revealing.

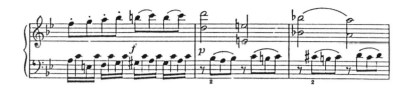

Example 8.6

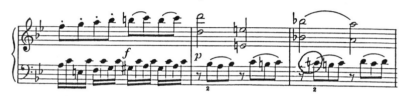

Example 8.6A

A final example (8.7) occurs in the coda where one note, D flat, makes all the difference:

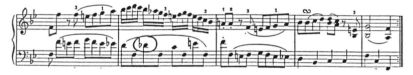

Example 8.7

If you go slowly and substitute a D natural as might be expected, it seems as if all the meaning has been taken out of it. If I heard that I might say "Oh! That's very nice; that's fine." But Mozart's compositional process sets up a context of highly sensitized awareness so that when one unexpected chromatic note appears we feel that our emotional stability has been seriously threatened for an instant and then recovered. That one note produces a moment of doubt which in its immediate resolution is infinitely consoling. I think that when we recall what all those people were saying about Mozart's performance there was something far more than just playing the keys under the cloth. He wasn't simply amazing them; he was touching them, too. I think that this is how he was doing it.

REFERENCE

Deutsch, O. (1965), *Mozart: A Documentary Biography*. Stanford, CA: Stanford University Press.

9

Mozart in D Minor—or, The Father's Blessing; The Father's Curse

Stuart Feder, M.D.

The central issue and core theme of applied psychoanalysis has consistently been the transformation of mind to art (Feder, 1993a). As an interdisciplinary endeavor, it aspires to the clarification of the "mysterious leap" from private, abstract mentation to a public, concrete, and formal work of art, whatever its medium.

Early in the history of applied psychoanalysis, biography became the point of entry into the mental life of the artist and interpreted content, particularly that related to fantasy, central to the understanding of content in art. Although rarely spelled out, this was viewed as not merely analogous to the content of mental life but as a true psychic derivative which resulted from a special kind of displacement. In the 1980s sophisticated studies such as those of Liebert (1983) demonstrated competence in the field of application as well as sensitivity to an ever-widening range of psychoanalytic possibilities which included issues of form. Only more recently has the strictly formal element in art in its relation to psychoanalysis received specific treatment in the work of Rose (1980) and Spitz (1985).

When the aesthetician, Walter Pater, wrote (1873) "all art constantly aspires toward the condition of music" (p. 111), it was this formal element which he sought to discriminate from among those representational elements which tend to be viewed as the "content" of a work of art. Indeed it is largely owing to the absence of such apparently representational features in music that there have been so few psychoanalytic contributions. What has been written of quality has tended to be about the *psychology* of music in general as opposed to articles on specific composers or, rarer still, specific works. Articles by Kohut (1957), Kohut and Levarie (1950), and Nass (1971) may be cited. Articles such as Noy's, which deal with formal elements in music, were by far the exception (1990).

In a series of contributions from 1978 to 1987 (Feder, 1978, 1980a,b, 1981a,b, 1982a,b, 1987) I attempted to explore the life and work of two composers, using the music itself as data to be related psychoanalytically to the mental lives of its creators. Accordingly, formal features were necessarily considered in terms of possible meanings and functions. The point of entry into mental life was biographical, and the composers selected, Gustav Mahler (1860–1911) and Charles Ives (1874–1954) were both born in the second half of the nineteenth century. They were thus part of a Romantic zeitgeist in which the boundaries of art and autobiography were frequently blurred, at times quite consciously—even self-consciously.

At the opposite end of the scale, or close to it, is the case of Mozart. Any consideration of his music throws into relief certain problems in the practice of psychoanalytic biography with specific reference to interpretation and the content–form issues. To many, Mozart is the exemplary musician of western civilization, his music not only representing the essence of the Viennese classical period but in many ways defining the way we think about "pure" music. Typical of this point of view is Paul Henry Lang (1963) who wrote: "The elements of Mozart's greatness are beyond analysis and discussion. Other great musicians can be discussed, but *his music does not offer an opening*—it is pure, unbroken, finished to the very end . . ." (p. 12; emphasis added). An intellectual challenge to this point of view was issued by the philosopher-musicologist-sociologist Theodor Adorno (1976) when he asserted: "Of all the tasks awaiting us in the social interpretation of music, that of Mozart would be most difficult and the most urgent" (p. 70). This is equally true with regard to psychoanalytic studies of music.

In recent years several music scholars have in fact sought a point of entry through the music into aspects of the life of Mozart, with specific reference to formal elements. Two, McClary (1985) and Subotnik (1991), both influenced by Adorno, have attempted interpretation in the spheres of social and historical aspects of Mozart's life, as opposed to individual mental life, let alone intrapsychic conflict. Others, however, notably Treitler (1989) and Epstein (in press) have dealt with what we must consider to be representations of conflict and affect in the music itself.

Accepting the challenge of the possible application of a psychoanalytic approach, I have been interested in studying certain formal elements in the music of Mozart against the background of biographical documents in which particular aspects of psychic conflict are revealed. Such formal features of the music may be viewed as apparently content-free "containers" or "organizers" for musical thought. One category consists of Mozart's use of specific tonalities. In what follows, I propose specifically to consider Mozart and the key of D minor. At the core of the associated mental conflict is Mozart's relationship with his father, Leopold Mozart, and the central biographical document, the remarkable body of correspondence between father and son (Anderson, 1938).

MOZART, FATHER AND SON

Of all the children born in the year 1756 few could have been as fortunate as Johannes Chrysostom Wolfgangus Theophilus Mozart. There are three important reasons, first that of survival itself: Mozart, the result of his mother's seventh pregnancy, was only the second and final surviving child. A sister, called Nannerl, was born four-and-a-half years earlier. His unsurpassed gift is the obvious second reason, the powerful genetic endowment which was at once an essential part of creative equipment and the foundation for character.

The third felicitous circumstance of Mozart's birth was to have Johann Georg Leopold Mozart for a father. The details of Leopold's life as well as Wolfgang's early life within the family are considered elsewhere in this volume. In what follows, only certain aspects of the relationship between son and father will be highlighted. But by the time Wolfgang was 7 and touring the world's capitals with his family, he was already an accomplished musician—not exclusively the result of a native talent: Leopold had been teacher and guide as well as father. By then, Leopold's life was deeply enmeshed with that of his son. He had been the boy's collaborator in virtually every one of Wolfgang's early compositions. But more than that, he was curator of body and soul. No detail of life escaped him and little was beyond his sphere of attempted mastery if not control.

If Leopold came too close as mentor, advisor, secretary, and valet—later as self-appointed best friend—the relationship served the
function of providing a model for as much good sense as Mozart was
ever likely to acquire. However, the complex bond that this closeness
engendered was one with which Mozart struggled during the course
of his entire life.

And further, if Leopold also served as impresario and entrepreneur for the child prodigy it was not necessarily exploitation. Leopold
was in a position not only to know full well exactly what both parent
and child had on their hands in these unusual talents, but the limited
options that lay open for their exercise in the future. In addition,
childhood, as we know it, did not exist at that time which is not to say
that there failed to be distinct developmental phases. For example,
Mozart retained a kind of access to the infantile which, going beyond
the normal, was in many ways characteristic of persons of genius as
described by Greenacre (1957). While this manifested itself superfi-
cially in a kind of childlike playfulness, sometimes with the scatological
content which was expurgated from early biographies, there was a
deeper, powerful, and in some ways more malignant force which
bound him to his father.

The well-known Mozart legend that has the child saying: "After
God, Papa" reveals precisely what the ever-present child-in-the-man
would have to contend with forever. And for his own part, Leopold
did not forego the role. His own identification with God—dormant
since he renounced the priesthood but exercised in his style of fatherhood—was too compelling. Rationalized, it became his duty as God's
missionary to convince the world of the "miracle" in which he knew
he played no small part; the moreso, he felt, in an age when people
no longer believed in miracles. "Therefore," he concluded, "they must
be convinced" (Sadie, 1980).

A man of the Enlightenment nonetheless, and author of the definitive *Versuch einer gründlichen Violinschule*, Leopold's interests were
wide. He owned not only a piano, violins, and other instruments, but
instruments of science as well, a microscope and two telescopes. To
have a fascination with music, as he did, and to possess the most
unimaginably supple *human* instrument could have been too seductive
for the Pygmalion in him. The temptation is that of playing so rare
a human instrument as if it were an extension of parts of oneself
rather than a separate human being whose autonomy must be respected, and who must, in fact, eventually separate. Happily, whatever

thrust there may have been in this direction must have been modified by both parents' sensitivity to the child. More than this, it would have been countered by a rapidly developing *artistic autonomy* in the growing Mozart, one which not only far outstripped the development of other psychological functions but contributed positively to their development.

Documentation has come down to us in an uncommon form, the 1765 equivalent of psychological testing! The Mozart family spent fifteen months in England during the course of a grand European tour which lasted three-and-a-half years, Wolfgang then being between the ages of 7½ and 11. In London he was examined by the philosopher Daines Barrington of the Royal Society, who later presented his findings in the form of a paper to the Society. Dr. Barrington's report consists of a history, gathered from several sources, along with his findings. Expectably, Leopold was present during the session. We know that because one of the tests devised by Barrington was to present the boy with a manuscript score which he could not possibly have seen before, which also contained some parts in the contralto clef. After Wolfgang played the introductory *Symphonia* flawlessly, he immediately turned to sing the upper voice part, leaving the lower one to Leopold. Barrington noted that the father "was once or twice out, though the passages were not more difficult than those in the upper one; on which occasions the son looked back with some anger pointing out to him his mistakes, and setting him right" (Daines Barrington's Report on Mozart, November 28, 1769, in Deutsch, 1965, pp. 95–101). Thus the 8-year-old who might otherwise feel quite attached, dependent, and obedient could frown disapprovingly at the flawed professionalism of his father who couldn't read music fast enough in the unfamiliar clef. It was precisely this kind of self-confidence which Leopold had nurtured that became ensconced in character. Born of artistic autonomy and generalized, it was among the elements that eventually fostered independence in composition and in psychological separation as well.

Leopold himself could be obedient and even subservient. Enlightenment aside, it was part of both the religious and temporal worlds in which he lived. He seemed comfortable in both, and if the *ancien regime* demanded compliance, he also knew how to maneuver within the system. Naïveté was not one of his traits and he showed considerable political skill. His demands on his son for obedience had multiple sources. It should be borne in mind that Leopold was a composer as well. This was a source of considerable esteem, and if residues of latent competition with his son did not linger, there was at least a sense of entitlement for services rendered and sacrifices made. At length he would prove punitive and beyond that he would carry a bitterness to the grave.

Leopold attempted to inculcate into Wolfgang submission to the will of God, to the will of the Emperor, and, above all, to the will of Count Colloredo, the Archbishop of Salzburg, who put bread on the table. Subsumed under all was obedience to the father. With regard to God and Emperor (and, *pari passu*, royalty in general) he met with considerable, if only formal, success. Wolfgang knew very well how to handle himself skillfully in their presence when he wanted to, mouthing "Your Majesties" and writing "Will of God" with equal facility whatever his inner feelings. He had learned these evasions from a master, and in time would turn the technique against Leopold himself. As for the Archbishop, open conflict with him proved to be Leopold's Waterloo as Colloredo became a transference figure for Wolfgang in the adolescent struggle for autonomy.

The biographical detail from the period of Mozart's Paris journey and death of his mother in 1778, to his definitive move to Vienna and marriage in 1782 is well known and will not be recounted here. It is a human story of maternal bereavement and restitution; of paternal conflict, yet identification; of rebellion and of personal and artistic growth. Back in Salzburg in 1781, at the penultimate moment of separation from Leopold, Mozart had hardly returned amiably to that dependency to which he had been trained. Rather, he perceived the potential for personal bondage—and perhaps creative as well—in his relationships with both Leopold *and* the Archbishop. Certainly, the psychological pathway for displacement between the two was well established, resentment for the Archbishop informed by Mozart's rage at the continuingly infantilizing Leopold. The provocation which earned Mozart dismissal accompanied by the legendary "kick on my arse . . . by order of our worthy Prince Archbishop" (Blom, 1935, p. 104) was an enactment of desperation not without insight. It was a kick that was prophetic. From this point on, not only would Mozart make choices which had an element of self-punishment for his revolt against the father, but he would at length re-create the ultimate crime of patricide, as well as its punishment, in *Don Giovanni.*

Mozart's move from the Archbishop's quarters in Vienna, to the home of the Webers with whom he boarded, was the turning point.

He was taken with Constanze Weber, having been spurned earlier by her older sister, Aloysia. The dream of earning his own living as a free artist in Vienna was countered by agitated letters from Leopold who continued to attempt to direct every detail of his son's life from afar. This met with equally frantic attempts on Wolfgang's part to appear to be obedient to his father while dealing at the same time with his need to separate. The need had by now became urgent, inextricably entwined as it was with the imperative to seek restitution for the loss of family life: not only that relating to his mother, but now the loss of Leopold as well.

The result was courtship and engagement to Constanze over the protests and admonitions of Leopold; even the withholding of the paternal blessing. Leopold's grudging consent arrived from Salzburg the day after the wedding in August of 1782. The groom was 26, the bride 20. On the wedding certificate Wolfgang used neither the baptismal string of names given to him by his parents nor the Italian, French, or romanized version of his "love-name," Gottlieb, which he had tended to use since the age of 14: Amadeo, Amadée, or Amadeus. Rather he signed it, Wolfgang Adam Mozart taking for himself the name God gave to his first human creation as he entered the estate of marriage.

MOZART IN D MINOR

Musicologists have observed changes in Mozart's employment of minor keys after 1778, the year of the pivotal Paris journey although very generally, Mozart did not favor minor keys (Hildesheimer, 1983). Martin Chusid (1967) in a study of Mozart's dramatic music noted that of four hundred individual operatic numbers, only thirty-four were minor, five in D minor. A comparable situation was found to obtain for the purely instrumental works. In the vocal music Chusid observed that the D minor numbers related "to a single dramatic situation: vengeance, either administered by the gods or sworn with the gods as witnesses" (p. 89).

Stylistically two juvenile pieces in D minor were written in imitative and conventional baroque style, although their texts do indeed relate to the literary theme of vengeance. The oratorio, *Betulia Liberata* of 1771, relates the tale of Judith and Holofernes in which Judith, in a lengthy recitative in D minor, describes her beheading of the Assyrian general in considerable clinical detail. In the D minor finale of *Thamos, King of Egypt* (before 1776?) angry gods have struck the blasphemer with a lightning bolt. Such early creative experiences may have served as the foundry for later works in which literary themes and related private fantasy became associated within a particular technical framework; here, the tonality of D minor. These efforts, however, were a far cry from such dramatically expressive D minor works as Electra's aria in *Idomeneo* of 1781 and the late Queen of the Night aria from *The Magic Flute* fully a decade later. It was this decade, of course, that spanned the Viennese years, from the time Mozart left Salzburg in 1781 to his death in 1791.

We will now consider this period and its trail of instrumental *and* vocal D minor works in their biographical context. They track Wolfgang's actual, adult relationship with Leopold in a significant way: All are related to the father, fathering, or fatherhood. Their psychological underpinnings may be said to reside in Mozart's mental representation of the father with all its imaginative derivatives and related fantasies.

The period was ushered in by the composition of *Idomeneo* in the fall of 1780, Mozart proceeding to Munich in November. A copious correspondence ensued between father and son, since not only was Leopold still very much collaborator and critic but functioned here as intermediary with the librettist, Abbate Varesco. Meanwhile, Mozart's erstwhile beloved Aloysia married in October. The lack of mention of this is, of course, consistent with Wolfgang's tactical handling of his father, although it is possible that letters may have been lost. Any sense of aggression or anger is confined to coded remarks about the Archbishop, one of which spells out his name in a scatological acronym (Anderson, 1938, p. 672). Such references may have served as displacement as well, screening Mozart's anger at both his controlling father and the woman who betrayed him in fantasy by choosing another man. Electra's aria ("Tutte nel cor vi sento . . ."), written during this period, may be justly called Mozart's most vivid representation of an insanely furious affect. Like the chorus fleeing from the avenging monster at the end of the second act ("Corriamo, fuggiamo . . ."), it is in D minor.

A curious behind-the-scenes drama took place in technical discussions between Wolfgang and Leopold about how the "subterranean voice" of the avenging god should be depicted musically. Leopold had some quite definite ideas of a somewhat excessive, melodramatic nature—a flaw in his own compositions was his naturalistic bent. Mozart asked his father to "consider it carefully . . . and remember that the voice must be terrifying—must penetrate . . ." but if too prolonged "mean[s] nothing." He himself favored the brief presentation which prevailed, noting, "If the speech of the Ghost in *Hamlet* were not so long, it would be far more effective . . ." (Anderson, 1938, p. 666). Mozart had recently seen a performance of *Hamlet* and had been much impressed by it. But unlike Hamlet himself, Mozart proved to be decisive in dealing with whatever wishes existed in ridding himself of either of his fathers—Leopold or the Archbishop. It was the following May of 1781 that the final break with the Archbishop took place as a result of which Mozart settled in Vienna. The following year he married Constanze.

In June of 1783 Wolfgang wrote to Leopold asking him to be godfather and namesake to their first child, whose birth was now imminent. On the 17th Constanze was in labor with their first son, Raimund Leopold. Wolfgang, in the adjoining room, was working on the second movement of his D Minor Quartet (K. 421) of the set dedicated to Haydn. Writes the critic Eric Blom (1935): "one can understand that a work with so sinister a feeling in the first movement and so tender a note in the second should come of this unnatural occupation; but how a whole quartet could turn out so faultlessly organized at such a time passes all conception" (p. 122).

The infant died two months later while boarding with a wet nurse during the couple's first visit back to Salzburg, for the purpose of reconciliation. The visit was far from successful, their reception by both Leopold and Mozart's sister, Nannerl, was cool at best.

The ice, if not broken, was at least traversed, and a return visit was planned by Leopold in order to see first-hand what life was like in Vienna for the young Mozarts. Leopold remained with them between February and April of 1785. Among the works composed in anticipation of his visit was the *D Minor Piano Concerto* (K. 466) which Leopold heard and commented upon favorably in a letter to Nannerl who remained in Salzburg. Despite the wounds which Leopold continued to nurse, a degree of rapprochement was effected during this visit. Certainly Leopold's "miracle" was fully in evidence as Joseph Haydn himself told Leopold at a performance of the quartets Mozart had dedicated to him: "I tell you before God, and as an honest man, that your son is the greatest composer I know, either personally or by name; he has taste, and apart from that the greatest science in compo-sition" (Blom, 1935, p. 129). But Leopold, who may well have felt that he had sacrificed all for this son—including his own career as he saw it—was no longer the miracle's curator.

Tension between father and son next surfaced the following year when Leopold categorically refused to care for his two grandchildren while Wolfgang pursued what he considered to be promising possibili-ties in England, the country he had longed for ever since the happy journey of his youth. His father's letter was, in Leopold's own words "forcible and instructive," finally inspiring obedience, he hoped, on his son's part (Anderson, 1938, p. 902). In the absence of a reliable familial baby-sitter, the 30-year-old Wolfgang felt obliged to remain in Vienna, although shortly thereafter he made a famous and highly gratifying trip to Prague. There he received the commission for a new opera planned for the next autumn. He hastened home to con-sult with the librettist, Lorenzo Da Ponte, who suggested the subject of Don Juan. Mozart was to make it his own, however. In his hands it became the ultimate oedipal opera from its opening with Don Gio-vanni's violent possession of the woman and his murder of the man to whom she was most deeply attached, her father; to the Don's fla-grantly immoral, libertine, and provocative acts; to his arrogant chal-lenge to the ghost of the man he slew; and finally, to his punishment and retribution, drawn to hell by the father's hand.

In an anecdote from childhood, Mozart's ambivalence toward Leopold is revealed as the child, kissing Leopold goodnight, would tell him that when he became old he would keep him forever in a glass case (Blom, 1935, p. 10). In *Don Giovanni* the glass case of child-hood fantasy became transformed in the mind of the artist to the grave from which the father's ghost emerged. Never, in fact, would he quite find rest in the composer's mind. The central key of the entire music drama is D minor.

The portentous chords with which the overture begins are the same that recur in the final act when the ghost of the Father appears at Don Giovanni's door: "Don Giovanni, a cenar teco m'invitasti e son venuto" [. . . invited by thee behold me here as directed]." Six times Don Giovanni refuses to repent as several keys are traversed in the music, and we are returned at length to D minor as the Don is con-signed to the flames.

But it was *Leopold* who died in 1787, the very year Mozart was working on *Don Giovanni*: He died in May and the opera received its premiere in Prague in October. Mozart himself had four more years to live, a period which was productive of more of the finest of his mature works, including three more operas, *Cosi Fan Tutte*, *The Magic Flute*, and *La Clemenza di Tito*. There was never a creative decline although the years that followed were attended by a decline of health and economic circumstances.

Mozart neither lived a pauper in his last years nor did he die one (Braunberens, 1986). But the style of life he attempted to lead as a free artist in a musical world in transition left him far from secure. He had never achieved the protection and support of a patron, even when he apparently sought one. Perhaps this was the fate of his struggle with Leopold as a result of which, on the other hand, he did not have to submit to the demands and whims of a patron, nor the control. At the same time, the move to Vienna had put him in the mainstream of musical commerce which enriched his music in a way comparable to the earliest journeys with Leopold. But more than that, whatever inner psychological independence he achieved in the separation fostered the continued maturation of a rare gift. No longer the Wunderkind, he became the master.

In 1791, "a gaunt messenger dressed in grey" came inquiring if Mozart would undertake to write a mass for the dead (Blom, 1935, p. 158). Mozart agreed to a not-unaccustomed business arrangement, after consultation with Constanze. The messenger appeared twice more during the course of the year, which was Mozart's last. Actually, the messenger was an emissary of a Count Walsegg, a recently be-reaved music lover who also liked to pass off the music of others as his own. A combination of the messenger's actual, becloaked, and somewhat sinister appearance and Mozart's toxic mental state as he became mortally ill later in the year, would have fostered a fantasy that this was indeed the messenger of death. When Mozart finally took to his bed, never to recover, the manuscript of the *Requiem* lay on the quilt. Like others of the compositions which track Mozart's mental trend of the father, it is written in the key of D minor.

DISCUSSION

Psychologically, perhaps the greater "miracle of Salzburg" was that Mozart was able to leave Salzburg and Leopold at all. Rather, the opposite was the case; separation became imperative and was carried out by Mozart with a mixture of mature ingenuity and adolescent bumbling. The sense of restrained urgency revealed in his letters of the time suggest what might have been at stake for him: nothing less than body and soul (Feder, 1993b)! As the year of his marriage approached he begged his father:

> But I entreat you, dearest, most beloved father, to listen to me. I have been obliged to reveal my intentions to you. You must therefore allow me to disclose my intentions to you, my reasons, which, moreover, are very well founded. The voice of nature speaks as loud in me as in others, louder, perhaps than in many a big lout of a fellow . . . [Anderson, 1938, p. 784].

Perhaps, too, the nature of the music that he would continue to compose also hung in the balance. One may only speculate as to what the music of the final decade would have been like had Mozart not been capable of leaving Leopold. This is more than beside the point. Rather, the need and the capacity to leave reflected aspects of ego strength which were intricately tied up with the musical gift. These gifts had been nurtured by Leopold, who was not prepared for what for him, was its bitter consequence. Further, it was in part Mozart's identification with his father that enabled him to even conceive of such a step, let alone negotiate it and survive, containing at the same time his "kick-in-the-arse" fury. Regrettably, he lacked Leopold's gift for the management of a career.

More than this, the early dyadic relationship with the father, inextricably interwoven as it was with music, failed to prevail as the dominant motivating factor in Mozart's life. It is here that the modest and biographically silent mother, Anna Maria Pertl Mozart, very likely exerted a tacit influence. Unlike other intense father–son relationships in art—Franz Kafka (Blos, 1985) and Charles Ives (Feder, 1992) may be mentioned—the triadic, or oedipal constellation supervened and, in the final analysis, prevailed. Some Mozart biographers question the appropriateness of Mozart's choice of Constanze as a marriage partner, reflecting in some measure Leopold's view and perhaps his wish as well. Psychologically speaking, she may have been a logical if not perfect choice: She was evidently a good-looking and sexy young woman, fun-loving with a down-to-earth capacity for intimacy.

But earlier and unresolved dyadic issues dogged Mozart to the end, one of which was the persistent wish for the father's blessing.

Blos (1985) writes of a point at the termination of adolescence "when the father's affirmation of the manhood attained by his son, conveyed in what we may call the father's blessing of the youth's impatient appropriation of adult prerogatives and entitlements, reaches a critical urgency" (p. 11). While adolescence may not have been literally identical in the eighteenth and twentieth centuries, arguably, the underlying principles in developmental goals and accomplishments remain constant. The father's final blessing, which may have served to ease, although not resolve, residues of early and persistent paternal conflict, was alternately withheld by Leopold or only grudgingly granted.

With regard to the key of D minor, works in this tonality appear to cluster around issues biographically related to father, fathering, and fatherhood and affects of rage and vengeance for transgressions against God and father. Nothing less than life and death hover in the balance and the final D minor work is the *Requiem* mass. This key is viewed as both a formal element, musically speaking, and one of elusive content: a musical idea or an aural image in the mind of the composer, which had become associated over the course of time with a complex of actual and mental events. To use a twentieth-century computer analogy, the tonality itself may have served as a file long since available in creative work which could be opened and added to under certain circumstances.

As for the *Requiem* itself, behind the discharge of a commission, for which Mozart had already been paid, was the discharge of another debt. The fantasied transgressions of the child, the enduring Don Giovanni-in-the-man, had to be paid for. A life was owed the father who had made him; the father whom the child in fantasy, and later the man in life and in art, had gotten rid of. Whatever else, the writing of the *Requiem* is an act of expiation representing a wished-for reunion with God and father. Musically, there is no question that Mozart intended his last notes to be in the key of D minor.

REFERENCES

Adorno, T. (1976), Introduction. In: *Sociology of Music*, trans. E. B. Ashton. New York: Seabury Press.

Anderson, E., ed. (1938), *The Letters of Mozart and His Family*, 4th ed. New York: W. W. Norton, 1989.

Blom, E. (1935), *Mozart*. Master Musicians Series. London: J. M. Dent.
Blos, P. (1985), *Son and Father—Before and Beyond the Oedipus Complex*. New York: Free Press.
Braunbehrens, V. (1986), *Mozart in Vienna, 1781–1791*. New York: Grove/Weidenfeld.
Chusid, M. (1967), The Significance of D Minor in Mozart's Dramatic Music. In: *Mozart Jahr-Buch*, Salzburg Mozarteum, pp. 87–97.
Deutsch, O. E. (1965), *Mozart—A Documentary Biography*. Stanford, CA: Stanford University Press.
Epstein, D. (in press), *The Sounding Streams: Studies of Time in Music*. New York: Schirmer Books/Macmillan.
Feder, S. (1978), Gustav Mahler, Dying. *Internat. Rev. Psychoanal.*, Part 2. 5:125–148.
———— (1980a), Gustav Mahler Um Mitternacht. *Internat. Rev. Psychoanal.*, 7:11–25.
———— (1980b), Decoration Day: A boyhood memory of Charles Ives. *Musical Quart.*, 66/2:234–261.
———— (1981a), Charles and George Ives: The veneration of boyhood. *Annual of Psychoanalysis*, 9:265–316. New York: International Universities Press.
———— (1981b), Gustav Mahler: The music of fratricide. *Internat. Rev. Psychoanal.*, 8:257–284.
———— (1982a), Charles Ives and the unanswered question. *Psychoanal. Study of Soc.*, 10:321–351. Hillsdale, NJ: Analytic Press.
———— (1982b), The nostalgia of Charles Ives: An essay in affects and music. *Annual of Psychoanalysis*, 10:301–332. New York: International Universities Press.
———— (1987), Calcium light night and other early memories of Charles Ives. In: *Fathers and Their Families*, ed. S. Cath., A. Gurwitt, & L. Gunsberg. Hillsdale, NJ: Analytic Press, pp. 307–326.
———— (1992), *Charles Ives: "My Father's Song."* New Haven & London: Yale University Press.
———— (1993a), Promissory notes: Psychoanalysis and music. In: *Psychoanalytic Explorations in Music: Second Series*, ed. S. Feder, R. Karmel, & G. Pollock. Madison, CT: International Universities Press, pp. 3–19.
———— (1993b), A tale of two fathers, discussion of Robert L. Marshall, *Bach and Mozart: Styles of Musical Genius*. In: *Explorations in Music: Second Series*, ed. S. Feder, R. Karmel, & G. Pollock. Madison, CT: International Universities Press, pp. 171–177.
Greenacre, P. (1957), The childhood of the artist: Libidinal phase development and giftedness. *The Psychoanalytic Study of the Child*, 12:47–72. New York: International Universities Press.
Hildesheimer, W. (1983), *Mozart*, trans. M. Faber. New York: Vintage Books.
Kohut, H. (1957), Observations on the psychological functions of music. *J. Amer. Psychoanal. Assn.*, 1–4/5:389–407.
———— Levarie, S. (1950), On the enjoyment of listening to music. *Psychoanal. Quart.*, 19:64–87.

Lang, P. H. (1963), *The Creative Work of Mozart.* New York: W. W. Norton.

Liebert, R. (1983), *Michelangelo.* New Haven & London: Yale University Press.

McClary, S. (1985), A musical dialectic from the enlightenment: Mozart's Piano Concerto in G Major, K 453, Movement 2. *Cultural Critique,* Vol. 4, Telos Press, 1985, pp. 129–169.

Nass, M. (1971), Some considerations of a psychological interpretation of music. *Psychoanal. Quart.,* 40:303–316.

Noy, P. (1990), The development of musical ability. In: *Psychoanalytic Explorations in Music,* Vol. 1, ed. S. Feder, R. Karmel, & G. H. Pollock. Madison, CT: International Universities Press.

Pater, W. (1873), "The School of Giorgione." In: *The Renaissance.* New York: Random House, Modern Library.

Rose, G. (1980), *The Power of Form.* New Haven & London: Yale University Press.

Sadie, S. (1980a), Mozart, Wolfgang Amadeus. In: *The New Grove Dictionary of Music and Musicians,* Vol. 12, ed. S. Sadie. London: Macmillan, pp. 680–752.

———— (1980b), Mozart, Leopold. In: *The New Grove Dictionary of Music and Musicians,* ed. S. Sadie. London: Macmillan, pp. 675–680.

Spitz, E. H. (1985), *Art and Psyche.* New Haven & London: Yale University Press.

Subotnick, R. R. (1991), Evidence of a critical world view in Mozart's last three symphonies. In: *Developing Variations.* Minneapolis: University of Minnesota Press, pp. 98–111.

Treitler, L. (1989), Mozart and the idea of absolute music. In: *Music and the Historical Imagination.* Cambridge, MA: Harvard University Press, pp. 176–214.

10

The Three Trials of Don Giovanni

Thomas Bauman, Ph.D.

Three times in the course of *Don Giovanni*, Da Ponte and Mozart invoke the mechanism of the trial. Each of these invocations follows a single pattern: A misdeed of the "young and extremely licentious nobleman," as the libretto describes Giovanni, leads to a confrontation that takes on the form sanctioned by eighteenth-century cultural practice for the offense in question.

In the very broadest sense, the trial or test was a virtually inescapable element in the theaters and opera houses of eighteenth-century Europe. At least in those institutions with any pretensions to refinement, the purpose of a theatrical work or opera was not merely to entertain but to instruct. And in an almost endless variety of guises, the test served as an apt vehicle for the instruction of a work's protagonists and, often, its audience. Mozart's last three operas furnish good examples. The whole plot of *Così fan tutte* turns on an elaborate test of the fidelity of Dorabella and Fiordiligi (although the men are also enrolled in Don Alfonso's School for Lovers). In *La clemenza di Tito* the strategems that hatch from Vitellia's imperial ambitions test not only the limits of Tito's clemency, but also her own moral character and that of Sesto. The most obvious trials of all, one would think, are those undergone by Tamino and Pamina in *The Magic Flute*. But these, like the ones just cited, are trials in the broader sense—tests of self-discovery we might call them—in contrast to inquisitions instituted to safeguard a social order or to adjudicate rival claims.

We confront a real trial in the strict sense of the term in the first of the operas Da Ponte wrote with Mozart, in Act III of *Figaro*.

Marcellina and Bartolo have thrown in together; they hope to take revenge on Figaro and wreck his impending marriage to Susanna by pressing Marcellina's own trumped-up claim to his hand in a court of law. The actual proceeding doesn't get very far: It is mooted almost at once by the surprise revelation that Figaro is the son of Marcellina and Bartolo. What there is of an actual trial takes place offstage, as background preparation for the great sextet of filial recognition and reunion.

The three trials of Don Giovanni are an altogether different matter. Each one of them is an essential musical event in the opera, and each one is also deeply implicated in a series of problems that have persisted in critical understanding of this "opera of all operas." Criticism in our own age has preoccupied itself above all with the question of the work's generic identity (Bitter, 1961; Henze-Döhring, 1986). Is it a comedy or a tragedy, an opera buffa or an opera seria? While this concern may be symptomatic of what Carl Dahlhaus (1982) has wryly called "an epoch of extreme Nominalism," it also suggests our continued allegiance to a conception of art music as an autonomously evolving entity, best understood in terms of its own categories and materials rather than as the product of an engendering culture.

Both Mozart's own catalogue of his works and Da Ponte's published libretto classify *Don Giovanni* as a comedy, that is, as an opera buffa or dramma giocoso. For much of the nineteenth century, especially in Germany, these labels were simply ignored, and the opera was treated as a tragedy. Giovanni, as its central tragic figure, was often compared to Faust (Weinstein, 1959), and the majority of productions ended with his descent to hell, rather than with the moralizing of those he left behind that concluded the first production of the opera at Prague in 1787. Modern-day sympathy for these nineteenth-century readings fits hand in glove with our generic puzzlement, for the paradigm of opera buffa as we understand it simply cannot support what the figure of Giovanni has come to betoken in aesthetic practice. We may even incline, with Walter Benjamin, to the belief that this extraordinary opera "stands beyond the confines of genre" (Bitter, 1961, p. 135).

The binary polarity of buffa or seria could only arise because critics had come to conceptualize the opera's historical situation exclusively in terms of high art. Such was not initially the case, but the opera itself, by dint of its overwhelming popularity, crowded out of cultural consciousness the rich theatrical tradition of low-comic Don

Juan dramas in which its own roots were embedded, a tradition that was at its strongest in eighteenth-century Austria and southern Germany, and thus utterly familiar to every one of Mozart's contemporaries. During much of its history prior to *Don Giovanni*, the Don Juan theme was very closely associated with the popular theater, for which not only the categories of comedy and tragedy but also their emphasis on decency, order, and instruction were largely irrelevant. This became quite clear whenever writers sought to appropriate the legend into the legitimate theater. Molière was ambivalent about his *Dom Juan*, produced at Paris in 1665. It received only a few performances, and he elected not to include it in his published works. In 1736 Carlo Goldoni also attempted to create a respectable version for the Italian stage. Later on, in his *Memoirs* (1787), he set forth his opinion of the raw material he had to work with in this enterprise: "Everyone knows the bad Spanish play that the Italians call *Il convitato di pietra* and the French *Le Festin de pierre*. I have always regarded it with horror in Italy, and I could not understand how this farce sustained itself for so long, drawing crowds of people, and giving delight to a civilized nation. The Italian actors were astonished themselves, and either jokingly or by ignorance claimed that its author had made a pact with the Devil in order to sustain it" (cited in Heartz, 1990, p. 161). The actors Goldoni refers to are not those for whom he himself wrote, but ones involved with the improvisatory traditions of the *commedia dell'arte*. The very year in which Mozart and Da Ponte created their masterpiece, Goethe saw a version of the Don Juan tale on a popular stage in Rome. The old story kindled such enthusiasm that after a few weeks, in Goethe's words, "There was not a soul alive who had not seen Don Juan roasting in Hell and the Commendatore, as a blessed spirit, ascending to Heaven" (Kunze, 1972, p. 328).

These souls were not flocking to the theater for moral edification, nor were they coming away with any. Instead, the play gave them, as it had for centuries, precisely what was proscribed in well-bred comedies and tragedies—the grotesque, the farcical, and the terrifying. Neither Molière, nor Goldoni, nor Da Ponte and Mozart could remove these elements entirely from their versions.

What kind of character was Don Juan in the popular theater? By the standards of Molière or Goldoni he was no character at all but an archetype, the common property of a hundred different tellings of the old tale. Like other archetypes, he was as often known by a descriptive adjective as by his name: various versions call him The Depraved, The Licentious, The Dissolute, The Profligate, or even The Atheist. But unlike the case of his country cousin, Hogarth's Tom Rakewell of *The Rake's Progress*, in the eighteenth-century popular tradition no one thought to inquire very closely into how Don Juan got to be the way he is. He is a noble, to be sure, and every telling of the tale relies on the background of a court culture, if only as his socioeconomic base of operations. But Don Juan never reflects on his own behavior or his station, even though his intellectual superiority in dealing with those around him is never in doubt. He is always in action, heedless of any and all barriers to his pursuits.

This is the Don Giovanni we meet in Mozart's opera. A protagonist's first aria, by tradition, reveals the essence of his character. Giovanni's first solo utterance is "Fin ch'han dal vino," a frenetic anticipation of the madcap disorder that is to come in the ballroom scene. Similarly, it is a Giovanni in action that we meet the moment he sets foot on the stage. Mozart labeled the opening scene of the opera an introduzione. This type of ensemble was already well established in Italian opera buffa; its purpose was to create a preliminary tableau, setting the scene, mood, and ambiance against which the action proper could begin, usually in the recitative that followed immediately. Leporello's grouchy monologue, "Notte e giorno faticar," does so admirably, but with the appearance of Giovanni the plot suddenly is up and running at full speed. This was not Mozart's doing, nor Da Ponte's, but is there already in their model, Bertati's one-act *Don Giovanni o sia Il convitato di pietra*, produced at Venice eight months prior to the première of Mozart's own opera and set to music by Giuseppe Gazzaniga. It is also there in the countless Don Giovannis and Don Juans before them.

The introduzione, as an action ensemble, breaks some other precedents as well. For the only time in any Mozart opera, someone is murdered before the audience's eyes. What might have come as a shock in another opera, however, turns out once again to be a familiar ingredient in the Don Juan tradition. In almost all versions, the murder of the Commendatore sets a firm course through an ensuing picaresque series of amorous adventures toward Don Juan's final downfall. The duel dates back to the earliest stage version of the legend, *El burlador de Sevilla*, a play attributed to Tirso di Molina; it was published in 1630, during the high tide of the "cloak and dagger" dramas of the Spanish theater. The Spanish term for the genre is *capa y spada*, which actually means "cloak and sword." And it is by the sword that Mozart's Giovanni undergoes his first trial, the immediate and violent response to his first transgression in the opera.

Giovanni's misdeeds are all of a kind—those of the individual against order. Mozart and Da Ponte made Giovanni's threat to social stability musically and visually manifest in the opera's greatest scenic tour de force, the ballroom scene at the end of the first act. But why do Giovanni's offenses, exposed there in all their nakedness, require *three* trials in the course of the opera? Here it is important to recall another feature of the legend: Don Juan is not simply a seducer, he is also a hypocrite and a blasphemer. Three trials are needed because his sins challenge three essential social structures in eighteenth-century European civilization—family, class, and religion.

His attempt on Donna Anna's honor demanded by long-established protocol a trial by sword. An affront of this magnitude to a noble family had to be met immediately and forcefully. Here is what Abraham Bosquett wrote on the subject as late as 1817, in a guidebook published at London called *The Young Man of Honour's Vade-Mecum*: "I have never known a man whose heart was in the right place to bring an action for damages against another for seducing a beloved wife, a daughter, etc. For these and such like offences the law can make no adequate retribution—in such a state life is a burthen, which cannot be laid down or supported, till death either terminates his own existence or that of the despoiler of his peace and honour" (cited in Baldick, 1965, pp. 32–33).

Giovanni at first refuses to fight his elderly opponent, but the Commendatore's imputation of cowardice pricks him where he is most vulnerable: though he may resort to base stratagems to extricate himself from amatory difficulties, Giovanni never backs down from confrontations with other males. The duel lasts only a few bars, and is musically delineated by nothing more than a brief fanfare and some conventional sweeps in the strings. It is the death of the Commendatore that brings with it several remarkable musical events. The powerful diminished seventh chord that signals the fatal blow is the very sound to which the Commendatore as Stone Guest will return in the Act II finale. Here at the end of the introduzione, it leads directly into a hushed Andante—the "Moonlight Trio," as it is called, for by tradition the somber strains of the three men are usually sung with the scene bathed in the eerie rays of the moon. At such a moment, one would think, Giovanni must pause to reflect seriously, if only briefly, on his deed and its possible consequences. But instead he describes with almost clinical detachment the departure of the old man's spirit from his wounded breast, and he does so to a melody borrowed from Donna Anna's music earlier in the scene.

There are two other surprises. The conventional cliché uttered by a mortally wounded man on the Italian stage is "Son ferito," "I am wounded," and that is what Bertati's Commendatore sings. But Da Ponte has him sing instead "Son tradito," "I am betrayed." Betrayed by whom? This is the first hint in the opera of the otherworldly dimension that is never absent from the Don Juan legend. Have the heavens themselves betrayed the Commendatore? For Giovanni's sword to have carried the day in such an unjust cause, they must be seriously out of joint. One senses unfinished business, and at the end of the trio, Mozart with a single stroke imprints in our ears this out-of-jointness, an impression that we will carry with us through the intervening episodes to the final catastrophe. The stroke is as ingenious as it is simple: The Moonlight Trio does not end, it stops in midair. The cadence we anticipate in its final bar is diverted at the last moment away from its expected resolution.

Formally, this evaded cadence opens up the possibility of hearing the introduzione as part of a larger opening tableau, one incorporating the overture at its beginning and the recitative and duet of Don Ottavio and Donna Anna at its end. For it is only after Anna has wrested a solemn oath of revenge from Ottavio that the tonal closure sidestepped by the final bars of both the overture and the introduzione arrives at last with a return to the opera's keynote, first sounded at the beginning of the overture.

There may also be a deeper, metaformal meaning to the introduzione's evaded cadence. Don Juan, we have mentioned, is an archetype. In the modern, Jungian spirit of the term, this means that whenever this mythic figure appears, he actualizes a collective, preconscious disposition within each of us, a "deep structure" built into the very nature of our species. As an actualization of the Don Juan archetype, Mozart's Giovanni confronts us not with a well-defined character or even a theatrical type, but with a "collective symbol." Marie-Louise von Franz (1981) interprets Don Juanism as a manifestation of the *puer aeternus* syndrome, marked by narcissism and an unwillingness to accept or abide by the rules and responsibilities of an adult community. The original Don Juan of Tirso di Molina, still strong in the

Giovanni of Da Ponte and Mozart, embodies a variant of the *puer aeternus*, the archetype of the trickster, common to a broad spectrum of cultures and mythologies. "Trickster" is in fact one translation of the word *burlador* in the title of Tirso's play. As a trickster, Don Juan involves himself in an endless game of attraction and deception that is only incidentally sexual: Its real function is to put off his day of reckoning with the ordered world he continually challenges and subverts. When his servant asks him what he thinks of that impending day, Tirso's Don Juan replies "Qué largo me lo fiáis!" ("That's a long way off!"). In deceiving others, he deceives himself.

The archetypal nature of Giovanni as a trickster who delays confrontation with adult reality carries an important implication for the analysis of Mozart's introduzione. Jung himself sought to study archetypal manifestations in human experience through the psychoanalysis of dreams, for which he took the structure of a drama as his point of departure (Jacobi, 1959). The formal *Gestalt* he developed begins with an exposition, which establishes the scene and the chief characters. Next, a peripeteia urges the plot forward, weaving events and images together until a third section, the climax, is reached. While this concludes the action proper within the dream, a necessary fourth section follows, the lysis (literally, a "loosening"). It restores, resolves, or otherwise reconfigures the dream's problematic elements in an effort to point up the meaning of the preceding action for the dreamer's psyche.

Da Ponte's introduzione follows this four-part pattern closely, as does the scene from Bertati's *Il convitato di pietra* which he had taken as his direct model. Yet while the two librettos exactly parallel each other in this initial scene, important distinctions emerge when we look at the music of Gazzaniga and Mozart. Gazzaniga's setting, while respecting Bertati's four-part division with closed cadences, is far more interested in musical continuity and character-drawing than in articulating the action; his tonal plan, in fact, scurries back to the tonic just as the drama reaches its climax with the appearance of the Commendatore. This in effect reduces his lysis to a musical epilogue, much as we may still admire the dark turn to E flat minor with which he limns the death of the Commendatore.

Mozart used a parallel modal shift to tonic minor at the same spot, but the dramatic effect is far more powerful, for in each of the preceding three sections—exposition, peripeteia, and climax—he had worked to create a distinctive tonal and motivic character; further, he took care to place the highest degree of tonal and thematic instability in the climax, where it belongs. The lysis, in this scheme, functions just as Jung described it, as a point of psychic restabilization that at once concludes and reflects on the action preceding it. But the "Moonlight Trio's" final, thwarted cadence tells us that the opera's initiatory dream has *not* concluded: Giovanni does *not* respond to this brief window of opportunity; he does *not* reflect on the meaning of his actions, and the day of reckoning is once more put off. This act of delay and of self-deception that we witness on stage is underscored in our ears by Mozart's deceptive cadence. In consequence, we along with Giovanni are forced to carry this moment and its unresolved psychic meaning through the activities of the following day to the second nocturnal visitation of the Commendatore that concludes the drama.

Before Mozart the Don Juan legend, as we mentioned earlier, followed its own ways, which are those of neither comedy nor tragedy. One of these involves the hero's amorous pursuits: They were of no fixed number, nor did they have to follow one another in any sort of logical fashion. In fact, the less they did so, the more impressive the inevitability of the final reckoning. Critics of Mozart's and Da Ponte's opera frequently point out the looseness of the episodes between the death of the Commendatore and the graveyard scene, especially in the first half of the second act. Here they in effect catch the opera straddling two worlds as it seeks to mediate the Don Juan of the popular theater with the formal demands of cultivated sensibilities in the opera house.

Bertati had made only the slightest effort in this direction. His Donna Anna, for example, drops out of the story completely after her scene with Ottavio following on the heels of her father's murder. Da Ponte, by contrast, is at obvious pains to keep the theme of revenge that she embodies alive throughout the drama. He also reminds us of the divine protection that sanctions her enterprise when the three maskers kneel in prayer prior to the first great confrontation between Giovanni and his foes in the Act I finale.

Further, during all of the episodes, Da Ponte avoids any sugges-tion of rivalry between Giovanni's real or potential conquests, which was a common feature of earlier Don Juan dramas and operas. Elvira rescues Zerlina from Giovanni's clutches after the duettino, and Anna responds sympathetically to Elvira in the Act I quartet. During all of these various episodes, in fact, evidence is being gathered and weighed in preparation for Giovanni's second trial. His dealings with Zerlina and Donna Elvira, quite apart from his culpability in Anna's tragedy, show again and again his utter disdain for the duties and social bearing his rank imposes. Giovanni's offenses against class and society require a trial by jury—the great sextet that comes in the middle of Act II, at which all whom he has offended in the drama are present. Here, too, the trial offers a vehicle for dramatic surprise—at least for the jury—when the accused is unmasked as Leporello. Such a base deception confirms at once Giovanni's abdication of his claim to nobility as anything more than a personal advantage to be exploited without constraint.

This is, of course, not a literal trial like the one in *Figaro*. In the ballroom scene Giovanni's guilt had already been exposed to everyone. But the sextet does carry earmarks of the kind of swift and pitiless justice meted out by the Venetian courts, which Da Ponte no doubt remembered vividly from his youth in and around Venice. Donna Anna and Don Ottavio, in their sober mourning garb, act as accusers, while Donna Elvira takes the part of attorney for the defense. Ottavio does not deign to offer Giovanni the opportunity to which his rank entitles him, namely a trial by sword, but is ready to run him through forthwith as a malefactor without privilege of station. It is at this point that Leporello sees the wisdom of abandoning his disguise.

Interpreters of *Don Giovanni* often invoke this and similar incidents in playing up the ties that link master and servant throughout the opera—ties that could hardly be made tighter than in Peter Sellar's production, where Giovanni and Leporello are played by identical twins. Yet in any but the most egalitarian culture the parallel between the two does not run very deep. Leporello, more than most cowardly servants, is a direct descendant of Harlequin, Hans Wurst, and their slapstick ilk, for it was one of them who, in the versions of the Don Juan story presented in the popular theater, always took the part of Juan's servant, and on whose *lazzi* the success of the piece largely depended. There is also in Leporello a little of Molière's Sganarelle, who ends the play the way Leporello begins the opera—with the complaint of a disgruntled employee. Sganarelle's immediate reaction on seeing his master dragged off to Hell is not to entertain any thoughts about the horrors of eternal damnation but to cry "My wages! My wages!"

No one is likely to make the mistake of admiring such a creature. His master, however, is another matter. The Don Juan archetype remains both recognizable and irresistible in his many manifestations throughout history because of a peculiarity in his nature that depends on no single social context—the resolute refusal of the *puer aeternus* to accept the consequences that society, whatever form it may take, prescribes for his actions. Leporello, on the other hand, is always worried about what will happen to him. He begins the opera wishing to play the gentleman as he stands guard outside Donna Anna's chamber; he ends it with the intent of seeking another master.

Nowhere is Giovanni's singular inability to yield to external constraints exposed on a grander scale than in his final confrontation with the Commendatore, the last of his three trials in the opera. Why the Don Juan legend favored the statue of the slain Commendatore as the vehicle for his undoing is an intriguing question. In the context of the opera, it could not be bettered, for the Commendatore's statue represents all three of the institutions against which Giovanni transgresses—family, class, and religion. As the Stone Guest the Commendatore is at once fallen kinsman, honored patriarch, and supernatural emissary.

What a happy thought on Mozart's part to link this scene musically with the death of the Commendatore by using the very sonority that marked Giovanni's fatal blow. But not simply because thereby he links crime and punishment. More importantly, that forceful chord connects the first glimpse we had received of Giovanni's incapacity for self-reflection with the final and grandest manifestation of that same trait. In theological terms, the verdict of this third, eschatological trial becomes inevitable through Giovanni's reckless exercise of contumacy and pride, the first and deadliest of the seven deadly sins. The Stone Guest demands that he repent, and fearlessly Giovanni refuses to do so.

In Jungian terms, this climactic scene tells us that the trickster archetype has so deeply embedded itself in Giovanni's ego that it is no longer to be forsworn even in the face of death. The pervasiveness of this archetype across human cultures attests to its primordial power. In the words of Joseph Henderson (1967) it offers "a kind of divinely sanctioned lawlessness that promises to become heroic" (p. 36). And that, in fact, is what it became when the nineteenth century transformed Giovanni from cynical outlaw into tragic outcast. Many modern readings of *Don Giovanni* share in the past century's admiration for his heroics in this final scene. But from the perspective of the Don Juan legend as Mozart's own audiences knew it, how could Giovanni do otherwise? How can a character incapable of self-examination repent of anything? There is something else at work in contemporary hero-worship of Giovanni, I am afraid, and that is our tolerance for (or even covert relishing of) the ungoverned workings of male sexual aggression. In modern criticism of Mozart's opera, this tendency's nadir was no doubt reached in 1977 with William Mann's perverse quip concerning Donna Anna, that "it would be beneficial to her personal growing-up if she had been pleasantly raped by Don Juan."

But quite apart from what such a remark tells us about its author, interpretations of this sort undervalue or ignore a lesson history has to teach us about Mozart's opera—its engagement with the complex counterclaims of a dual allegiance. On one side Mozart and Da Ponte had to reckon with the notoriety in which their theme was steeped through its long-standing cultivation in the popular theater. As mentioned earlier, that tradition is now lost to us. And it is lost precisely because Mozart and Da Ponte achieved what had been denied to the likes of Molière and Goldoni: They brought Don Juan fully into the pantheon of high art.

On the other side of the opera's dual allegiance looms a commitment that it shares with Mozart's other operas and with eighteenth-century theatrical ideals generally—a commitment to moral edification and aesthetic order. That is why the final sextet is there, to serve as the lysis that a structured society demanded when confronted with those who have not or cannot make their peace with its ways. And that is why the original title was not simply the name of the opera's notorious archetype, but *Il dissoluto punito, ossia Il Don Giovanni*—"The Dissolute One Punished, or Don Giovanni." The wording on which Da Ponte and Mozart settled is not simply another instance of the eighteenth century's fondness for double titles, but testimony to the complex and often opposing theatrical currents that were tributary to Mozart's greatest opera.

REFERENCES

Baldick, R. (1965), *The Duel: A History of Duelling*. New York: Clarkson N. Potter.

Bitter, C. (1961), *Wandlungen in den Inszenierungsformen des "Don Giovanni" von 1787 bis 1928: Zur Problematik des musikalischen Theaters in Deutschland*. Regensburg: Gustav Bosse Verlag.

Bosquett, A. (1817), *The Young Man of Honour's Vade-Mecum, Being a Salutary Treatise on Duelling*. London: C. Chapple.

Dahlhaus, C. (1982), Europäische Musikgeschichte im Zeitalter der Wiener Klassik. In: *Colloquium "Die stilistische Entwicklung der italienischen Musik zwischen 1770 und 1830 und ihre Beziehungen zum Norden" (Rom 1978)*. Laaber: Arno Volk-Laaber Verlag, pp. 1–20.

Goldoni, C. (1787), *Memoires de M. Goldoni pour servir à l'histoire de sa vie, et à celle de son théatre*, 3 vols. Paris: Veuve Duchesne.

Heartz, D. (1990), *Don Giovanni*: Conception and creation. In: *Mozart's Operas*, ed., with contributing essays, T. Bauman. Berkeley: University of California Press, pp. 157–177.

Henderson, J. L. (1967), *Thresholds of Initiation*. Middletown, CT: Wesleyan University Press.

Henze-Döhring, S. (1986), *Opera seria, opera buffa und Mozarts Don Giovanni: Zur Gattungskonvergenz in der italienischen Oper des 18. Jahrhunderts*. Laaber: Laaber-Verlag.

Jacobi, J. (1959), *Complex/Archetype/Symbol in the Psychology of C. G. Jung*, trans. R. Mannheim. New York: Pantheon Books.

Kunze, S. (1972), *Don Giovanni vor Mozart: Die Tradition der Don-Giovanni-Opern im italienischen Buffa-Theater des 18. Jahrhunderts*. Munich: Wilhelm Fink Verlag.

Mann, W. (1977), *The Operas of Mozart*. London: Cassell.

von Franz, M.-L. (1981), *Puer aeternus*, 2nd ed. Santa Monica, CA: Sigo Press.

Weinstein, L. (1959), *The Metamorphoses of Don Juan*. Stanford, CA: Stanford University Press.

11

Clues to Mozart's Creativity: The Unfinished Compositions

Robert L. Marshall, Ph.D.

Mozart has left a long trail of unfinished compositions. They come in all sizes and, variously distributed, at all times throughout the course of his creative life. But their extent and also their significance have been vastly underestimated. Between the 626 whole numbers of the *Köchel* catalogue, there are listings for more than 120 fragmentary pieces—that is, about one for every five completed works (Köchel, 1965, passim). But that number does not convey the full picture, since there are no fewer than thirty-three fragmentary works that have regular "Köchel" numbers—works like the *Requiem*, K. 626, and the C Minor Mass, K. 427. The number thirty-three, then, should really be subtracted from the 626 and added to the 120, bringing the proportions—in round numbers—to something like 600 to 150, or one fragment for every four completed works.

There are unfinished pieces in the "London Sketchbook" dating from the year 1764, when Mozart was 8 years old;[1] others continue to appear up to the very end with the *Requiem*. But the fragments are by no means evenly distributed throughout his life. The period of their greatest concentration is the fifteen months or so from the summer of 1782 to the late fall of 1783; this is the period following the premiere of *Die Entführung aus dem Serail*, and embracing both his

---

[1]See the three-measure sonata incipit in F, K. 15nn, the 12-measure fragment for a minuet in C, K. 15rr, and the 23-measure fragment of a fugue for four voices and continuo, K. 15ss, all in the new complete edition of Mozart's works: *NMA*, Vol. IX/ 27/1: *Klavierstücke. Die Notenbücher*, pp. 163, 166–168.

marriage to Constanze Weber and his subsequent return home to Salzburg. During this period there are traces of some thirty-two unfinished compositions. In contrast, for the entire early period—the fourteen years from 1764 to 1778—there are only some eighteen such documents altogether.

The years 1777 to 1779 are the critical years of Mozart's travels to Mannheim and Paris, the first extended journey without his father and one during which he experienced his first serious, and frustrating, love affair (with Aloysia Weber), along with continual professional disappointments in Paris, and, above all, the death of his mother there in early July of 1778. It should not be surprising, then, that the first notable concentration of significant unfinished works dates from this period and its aftermath. Among them we find a Singspiel (*Zaide*, K. 344/336b), a church piece (a 34-measure Kyrie fragment in E Flat, K. 322/296a, dated to early 1779 by Wolfgang Plath [see Plath, 1977, p. 170]), and a couple of remarkable concertos for multiple soloists (to which I shall return).

Mozart's first months in Vienna, beginning in March 1781, constitute another crucial turning point in his life. Once again the incompletion rate is high: During the following nine months, until the end of that year, there is one unfinished composition for every two completed works (6:12). And, once again, physical and emotional stress may hold the explanation. For this is the period just following the premiere of *Idomeneo*, which took place in Munich in January 1781. It was no doubt a time, then, like that following the premiere of *Die Entführung*, accompanied, we can be sure, by feelings of exhaustion, exhilaration, letdown. But this time, there were additional complications: Whereas the *Entführung* premiere was auspiciously followed in a month by Mozart's marriage to Constanze Weber, the premiere of *Idomeneo* was followed by six months of perpetual crisis, marked by the adjustment to life in Vienna and the intensely painful process of breaking with Salzburg. This was a process that, on the one hand, severely damaged Mozart's relationship with his father and, on the other, culminated not in marriage but rather in his ignominious "divorce," sealed with a kick to the seat, from the service of the Archbishop. Of course, this was a blessing only barely disguised, and Mozart knew it.

Over the course of the last eight years of his life, from 1784 on, Mozart managed to complete around 170 compositions, and managed *not* to complete some 60 further works, for a completion ratio of just over 3 to 1. Paradoxically, the year in which Mozart succeeded in finishing the greatest number of works—1788 (with some 35 completed compositions) is also the year that saw the greatest number of unfinished compositions: 16 (a ratio of 2:1).

Such statistics, of course, are only rough approximations. To begin with, many of Mozart's works, finished as well as unfinished, cannot be definitely dated. Moreover, even if we had precise dates for every composition, knowing the mere number of works composed in a given period of time still would not mean very much, since a little contredanse counts as "1" (e.g., K. 534), as much as does *Don Giovanni* (K. 527). And, indeed, the same point should be made about the unfinished works. They range in substance and content from the notation of a brief thematic idea of perhaps two or three measures to torsos of gigantic dimensions like the C-Minor Mass and the *Requiem*. While some fragments do no more than record the most embryonic of beginnings, others preserve nearly complete compositions—compositions that may even be performable in whole or in part. This is clearly so in the case of multimovement compositions—operas, concertos, sonatas, along with the Mass and the *Requiem*—in which some of the individual numbers were completely finished. There is one intriguing implication of this; namely, it is conceivable that a composition listed in the *Köchel* catalogue as an independent, single-movement piece—say, a rondo (or an andante) for flute (or violin, or piano)—may actually be the only finished movement of what Mozart originally had intended as a full-size concerto or sonata.[2]

Given their numbers, it is perhaps not very surprising that virtually every compositional genre is represented among the fragments: church music, German and Italian operas, concert arias, lieder, symphonies, along with chamber music, concertos, sonatas, and pieces for a colorful variety of instrumental combinations and soloists. The only form that is absent altogether is the opera seria. But this is readily explained: Mozart only took up the composition of a serious opera when he had received a firm contract—inevitably entailing a firm

---

[2]Conceivable examples are: the Adagio for Violin and Orchestra in E, K. 261; the Rondo for Violin and Orchestra in B Flat, K. 269/261a; the Andante for Flute and Orchestra in C, K. 315/285e; the Rondo for Piano in D, K 485; or the Adagio in B Minor, K. 540. Some of these, of course, could be substitution movements or additions to completed works. Of course, they could have been intended as independent items. Mozart, for example, describes K. 540 in his personal catalogue as "Ein Adagio für das Klavier allein"—suggesting that he considered it (at least at the time) to be an independent composition.

deadline on the one hand and a lucrative free, payable upon delivery, on the other. Works of that kind always took highest priority and were not readily set aside.

For the rest, we can detect several distinct patterns of distribution of the unfinished works among the various musical genres: There is a striking number of woodwind pieces. There are also a considerable number of unfinished church pieces—mostly the opening measures of Kyrie settings. As Tyson (1987) has shown, many of these date not from the Salzburg period but from the later Vienna years—from around 1788, to be precise (pp. 26–28). Similarly, there are numerous contrapuntal and fugal drafts which are now known to date from many different times, rather than to be concentrated, on the one hand, in the year 1770, in connection with Mozart's studies with Padre Martini, or, on the other hand, around the year 1782, when Mozart is supposed to have been strongly encouraged by both his wife Constanze and by Baron van Swieten to write fugues.[3]

From a purely musical point of view the most impressive collection of incomplete compositions, in my opinion, consists of the scores of some half-dozen instrumental compositions, mostly concertos, that had reached an advanced stage of formation before they were set aside. There can be no doubt that Mozart had been seriously committed to these pieces. They first appear in 1778 and reappear sporadically throughout the Viennese period.

CONCERTO FOR PIANO, VIOLIN, AND ORCHESTRA IN D, K. 315f

The first substantial torso belongs to a Concerto for Piano, Violin, and Orchestra in D Major which Mozart began in November 1778 in Mannheim on his journey home from Paris. The movement extends for 120 measures and is the longest incomplete work up to this time. Mozart intended it for himself and for the excellent Konzertmeister of the Mannheim Orchestra, Ignaz Fränzl (see Mozart's letter of November 12, 1778 [Anderson, 1938, p. 631]). The heading on the first

---

[3]According to Plath (1977), the canons, K. 73i, k. r-73x date from 1772, not 1770 (pp. 139–140); the fugue fragment, K. 401/375e dates not from 1782 but rather late summer 1772 (p. 161) and the fugue fragment 375g not from 1782 but rather 1777. According to Tyson (1987), the fugue fragment in G, K. 375d dates from 1785/86, not 1782 (p. 141).

page of the autograph manuscript is complete except for the date—an indication that Mozart was entirely confident about the prospects for the work.[4] The substantial opening ritornello is completely scored. (At 74 measures it is, as Levin [1970, p. 309] points out, the longest Mozartean concerto ritornello except for the C Major Piano Concerto, K. 503.) With the entry of the solo, however, the accompaniment is missing. The draft contains all or most of the thematic material of exposition; it also prepares for the modulation to the dominant, finally breaking off upon the arrival of the pivotal "V of V" (dominant of the dominant) harmony, the threshold of the new key.

The draft of the double concerto is an example of what may be called "block" or "sectional" composition. In each formal section Mozart first enters the melody or principal motivic parts, then the bass, then the filler parts. But he evidently proceeds then to finish the scoring of the drafted section before moving on to the next.

SINFONIA CONCERTANTE IN A MAJOR FOR VIOLIN, VIOLA, CELLO, K. 320e

Probably no more than a year later, sometime in the course of 1779, Mozart began to compose another multiple concerto, equally ambitious in scope and content, this time 134 measures in length: It was to be a sinfonia concertante for violin, viola, cello, and orchestra. It was written soon after his return to Salzburg, almost certainly at about the same time as the famous (and finished) Sinfonia Concertante in E Flat for Violin and Viola, K. 364/320d. It carries the adjoining number 320e in the latest *Köchel* catalogue.

As in K. 364, the viola part is transposed and intended for scordatura tuning, this time the transposition is a whole tone lower.[5] As in the double concerto, K. 315f, the opening ritornello is again completely scored; and once again, upon the solo entry the accompaniment is missing. This time, however, the solo parts are continued through the presentation of the secondary theme in the dominant

---

[4]The autograph is preserved in the Paris Bibliothèque Nationale Paris (Département de la Musique). A facsimile appears in *NMA* Vol. V/14/2, p. xviii; the fragment is transcribed on pp. 136–152.

[5]The fragment is in the possession of the Internationale Stiftung Mozarteum, Salzburg. A facsimile of the opening page appears in *NMA* V/14/2, p. xix, a transcription of the fragment appears on pp. 153–161.

and on to the soloists' closing theme. But the autograph breaks off before the cadence. In effect, however, the entire exposition has been notated: The arrival in the dominant this time is not only prepared, as in the concerto for piano and violin, K. 315f, but confirmed. But once again only the opening ritornello is fully scored. This is, then, another example of "block" composition.

The two concerto drafts share approximately the same formal, and even temporal, dimensions: In performance they each last about four minutes and continue to the change of key—stopping either at the threshold of the dominant or just crossing over it. This much of the form was evidently necessary, but also sufficient, to enable Mozart to fix and secure the viability of the new composition: defining and recording its principal thematic material along with its first significant modulation.

HORN CONCERTO IN E FLAT, K. 370b/371

There is an unfinished horn concerto dating from March 1781, the very beginning of the Vienna period. In this work Mozart's compositional procedures have changed in two respects. First of all, in contrast to the two preceding works, we now have material for two of the movements—both of them incomplete. Interestingly enough, the second movement, a rondo, is more complete than the first movement. Mozart, then, did not compose the movements in consecutive order; nor did he feel constrained to complete one entirely before moving on to the next.

It is difficult to know exactly how much of the first movement was written because the manuscript was cut up into numerous pieces—a dozen survive—and scattered around the world (see *NMA* V/14/5, p. xv). It is likely that the entire movement was drafted. The entire opening ritornello, the solo exposition, the dominant tutti, the brief development section, and most of the recapitulation are present. But, unlike the double and triple concertos, K. 315f, and 320e, the movement is nowhere fully scored. Only the principal parts are notated: melody-plus-bass, along with any motivically active accompaniment.[6]

---

[6]A facsimile of the surviving fragments of K. 370b, along with the autograph of the rondo, K. 371 (currently in private possession), are published in Pizka (1980), pp. 175–210.

The second difference between this draft and those of the two pre-Vienna concertos is this: In the earlier concertos Mozart apparently composed section by section in *blocks*. Here he is composing "horizontally" for the whole movement—a quite different compositional method.

The autograph for the second movement, the rondo, contains a heading with composer's name and the date: "21 de mars 1781." The presence of the date suggests that Mozart considered this piece in effect "composed," even though it was not completely scored. The movement is complete, however, in the sense that the notation reaches the end. It is in fact a combination of "block" and "horizontal" composition. The first two refrains of the rondo were completely scored; for the solo episodes and remaining refrains only the principal parts were written down.

CONCERTO FOR BASSET HORN IN G, K. 621b

Finally, there is a draft for a concerto for basset horn in G major, dating from 1787 or 1788 (for the date, see Tyson [1987, p. 35]). The draft stretches for a full 199 measures.[7] Although it is not completely notated, it may have been completely composed. First of all, the score breaks off at the end of a full double leaf, or bifolio (i.e., it may well have gone on). Second, it is virtually identical to the clarinet concerto, K. 622, which, of course, was completed—some three years later at the very end of Mozart's life.[8] The basset horn concerto can be taken as ideally representing the one pole of Mozart's compositional method: what I have been calling "horizontal" composition.

What all these compositions have in common, of course, apart from their outstanding quality, is their unusual scoring.[9] It is

---

[7]The autograph is in the possession of the Rychenberg-Stiftung, Winterthur. A complete facsimile is published in *NMA* V/14/4, pp. 165–176.

[8]From m. 180 on the notation of the bass line in the autograph is in A major, not G—an indication that from this point on Mozart was already conceiving the work in its later version for (basset) clarinet in A. As reported in *NMA* V/14/4, p. ix, these measures were added in a darker ink and sharper penpoint—perhaps only after a considerable interruption in time.

[9]There is also an unfinished quintet movement, in sonata form, for clarinet, basset horn, and strings in F, K. 580b, dating from 1789. It contains the music for the complete exposition to the double bar. Significantly, the opening section, through the arrival on the V/V is completely scored, while the remainder alternates between principal-part notation and full scoring—a combination, then, of "block" and "horizontal" composition (see *NMA* VIII/19/2, pp. 45–49).

clear—and sometimes specifically documented—that Mozart enthusiastically embarked on these compositions with a particular performer
(and perhaps even a particular performance) in mind. It is just as
clear that at some point his expectations were dashed, whereupon
Mozart set the piece aside—no doubt with the firm intention of resum-
ing work whenever an opportunity for a performance should present
itself.

Infinitely more, of course, could be said about Mozart's approach
to the task of composition. The principal tangible evidence bearing
on this question, as we have seen, is found in the autograph manuscripts of the music itself. But Mozart's letters, and also the observations of contemporaries, shed valuable light on the question, as well.
They testify, first of all, to the composer's need and desire for congenial circumstances, peace of mind, and adequate time to plan and to
contemplate. In a letter to his father from Paris, dated July 31, 1778,
Mozart declared, "I love to plan works, study, and meditate." Some
five years later, in a letter to his father from Vienna, dated July 5,
1783, he remarked, "I prefer to work slowly and with deliberation."
Mozart, however, rarely had these amenities—time least of all. He
composed at his legendary breathtaking speed out of necessity, not
inclination (see Marshall [1991, especially pp. 23–35], for additional
documentation bearing on Mozart's compositional process).

It is important, at all events, to distinguish the act of composing
from the act of writing down music. When the creative challenge
was relatively unproblematic—as, for example, in the composition of
simple recitatives (or ballroom dances)—then the act of conception
and the activity of writing for Mozart were virtually simultaneous. As
he reported to his mother from Milan on October 20, 1770, while he
was at work on his opera *Mitridate*, "I cannot write much [i.e., to her
at the moment], for my fingers are aching from composing so many
recitatives" (quoted in Marshall [1991, p. 30]). On the other hand,
Mozart's most significant works were the product of a shorter or
longer period of intense gestation: much, perhaps most of it, internal
rather than on paper, but no less intense for that. The grander the
conception, the more intensive the preliminary planning. According
to Mozart's widow, Constanze, "When some grand conception was
working in his brain, he was purely abstracted, walking about the
apartment, and knew not what was passing around" (quoted in Marshall, 1991, p. 30). But even after such internal preparation, there
was often the need for further working out, this time on paper. This

was notably the case when Mozart determined to raise the professional stakes for himself by publishing the composition. On such occasions, it would seem that the degree of his artistic self-criticism was heightened—or, perhaps, that the level of his personal self-confidence was lowered. This may help explain why the original manuscripts for compositions intended for publication—compositions, that is to say, that Mozart wished not only to present to the world but to preserve in relative permanence (in effect "for posterity")—by and large contain a significantly greater concentration of reworked and rejected passages than do the manuscripts of more "occasional" works (works like the concertos discussed here) that were intended perhaps for but a single performance. The heavily corrected manuscripts of the six celebrated string quartets Mozart was soon to publish—with a dedication commending these spiritual offspring to his revered older colleague, Joseph Haydn, and the "fruit," in Mozart's words, "of a long and laborious study"—provide perhaps the most dramatic example of Mozart exercising (or laboring under) his severest powers of self-criticism (see the facsimile edition, Tyson [1985]).

To return to the unfinished concertos. Our examination of the manuscript scores allows us to make one final general point about Mozart's compositional procedures. Whether he adopts the "block" approach typical of the pre-Vienna works or the "horizontal" approach of the Vienna period—and these, along with various mixtures and combinations of the two, represent his usual methods in the larger instrumental forms—it appears that the creative act was always driven forward, step by step along the unfolding form. Mozart, unlike Haydn, did not construct formal models or composition plans—plotting out in advance an opening idea in one corner of his score, a second theme somewhere else, or perhaps mapping the harmonic design of a development section by marking the cadence tones but leaving the connecting links (the transitions between these strategic points) to be added later on (Schafer, 1987). In a real sense, the act of composition for Mozart seems rather to have been a very fluent thing, indeed a "stream" of consciousness, or at least of artistic instinct wherein, as far as one can see, one thing (i.e., one musical idea), literally led to the next. After his death, Mozart's widow remarked (Mozart, C. 1799) that Mozart composed music as if he were writing a letter (col. 855). This may be what she meant.

REFERENCES

Anderson, E. (1938), *The Letters of Mozart and His Family*, 3rd ed., trans. E. Anderson. London: Macmillan, 1985.

Köchel, L. v. (1965), *Chronologisch-thematisches Verzeichnis sämtlicher Tonwerke Wolfgang Amadé Mozarts*. 7th ed., unrev., ed. F. Giegling, A. Weinmann, & G. Sievers. Wiesbaden: Breitkopf & Härtel.

Levin, R. D. (1970), Das Konzert für Klavier und Violine D-Dur KV Anh. 56/315f und das Klarinettenquintett B-Dur, KV Anh. 91/516c: ein Ergänzungsversuch. *Mozart-Jahrbuch 1968/70*:304–326.

Marshall, R. L. (1991), *Mozart Speaks: Views on Music, Musicians, and the World*. New York: Schirmer/Macmillan.

Mozart, C. (1799), Anekdoten. Noch einige Kleinigkeiten aus Mozarts Leben, von seiner Wittwe mitgetheilt. *Allgemeine Musikalische Zeitung*, 1: col. 855.

NMA (1955–), *Wolfgang Amadeus Mozart. Neue Ausgabe sämtlicher Werke. Neue Mozart Ausgabe*. Kassel: Bärenreiter-Verlag.

Pizka, H. (1980), *Das Horn bei Mozart. Facsimile-Collection*. Kirchheim: Hans Pizka Edition.

Plath, W. (1977), Beiträge zur Mozart-Autographie II. Schriftchronologie 1770–1780. *Mozart Jahrbuch*, 1976/77:131–173.

Schafer, H. A. (1987), *"A Wisely Ordered Phantasie": Joseph Haydn's Creative Process from the Sketches and Drafts for Instrumental Music*. Unpublished doctoral dissertation. Brandeis University, Waltham, MA.

Tyson, A. (1985), *The Six "Haydn" String Quartets. Facsimile of the Autograph Manuscripts in the British Library. Add. MS. 37763*, Intr. A. Tyson. London: British Library.

———— (1987), *Mozart: Studies of the Autograph Scores*. Cambridge, MA: Harvard University Press.

12

The Unfinished *Requiem*:
A Mystery That May Not Be Solved

George H. Pollock, M.D., Ph.D.

Biographers and autobiographers, at times, confuse fact, interpretation, and Procrustean wishes for simple explanations. This can result in distortions, false emphases, inaccuracies, and overt lies or omissions that reflect the authors' wish to present fact when they are actually writing fiction. The transferences and countertransferences of the writers become apparent as one is able to determine absolute facts that are agreed upon by reliable sources. In this essay, an attempt will be made to illustrate the above hypotheses focusing upon the story of a world famous musical creation, the *Requiem* of Mozart. Romanticized narrative intermixed with plausible snippets have perpetuated myths about the composer and his last uncompleted masterpiece that now can be more carefully examined for truth and inaccuracies. Some facts will never be known, some assumptions and assertions cannot be confirmed or refuted, but some of these can be tested against valid data and hence demonstrated to be true or false. In science, biography and autobiography, and the law, the burden of proof resides with the originator of the assertions. While philosophers argue about what is truth, in gross factual situations this may be less of a dilemma than is the case in less clearly defined situations.

I

Why the great emphasis on Mozart at this time? In 1991, the world celebrated the bicentennial of Mozart's death. This was an unusual event in that tradition emphasizes birthdays instead of death days, which are memorializations and usually associated with religious ceremonies. But Mozart's death was different. Many events—concerts, operas, radio and television programs—focused on this anniversary year. Intimately connected with Mozart's death was his famous *Requiem*, which he was working on at the time of his final illness, but never had the chance to complete.

Brown (1992) has correctly noted that the popularization of Mozart came from Shaffer's play, *Amadeus*, subsequently made into a movie shown worldwide. But as Brown indicates, Shaffer and the movie director, Milos Forman, stated, "we were not making an objective 'Life of Wolfgang Mozart' . . . [the play] was never intended to be a documentary biography of the composer and the film even less of one" (1992, p. 50). The tale was fictional and designed to entertain, not give an accurate historical picture of Mozart's death or the biography of his *Requiem*. "The caveats published with the stage play were never imprinted on celluloid; fiction was never segregated from truth" (Brown, 1992, p. 50).

Brown clearly emphasizes the difference between the fictional invention of Shaffer and Forman and the historical truth (a practice not unknown in other areas of biography, autobiography, court trials, etc.). Enough historical fact is utilized to give the product a coating of authenticity, but in order to be a productive marketing device the emphasis must be on appeal, rather than accuracy. The plot acquires a mysterious detectivelike focus. Motives are rearranged to suit the overall objectives of the promoters bent on entertaining the audiences even at the sacrifice of historical accuracy resulting in a leap from fact to fiction. Evidence does not support the narrative, although for purposes of amusement or other more serious goals, e.g., law suits, they suffice and are not seriously questioned. Thus Salieri did not poison Mozart; Mozart rarely drank to excess (Brown, 1992, p. 61); Mozart's extramarital sexual liaisons cannot be proven one way or another; the actual cause of his death can only be conjectured; a psychiatric diagnosis of cyclothymic disorder without psychosis is speculative; Mozart "was never poor by the standards of his time" (p. 64); "evidence does not support a negative view of Constanze" (p. 58) when she was married to him; and "Mozart's funeral and burial were arranged by the Baron Gottfried von Swieten, who adhered to the Josephian burial guidelines" (p. 65). In 1791, the burial experience of "the dumping of a bagged body into a communal grave . . . was the burial experienced by about 85 percent of Vienna's population. It was the norm, not an interment reserved only for the impoverished" (p. 65).

The serious student of musical creativity can ask, So what does this tell us about Mozart's creativity—how he got his ideas and how did he elaborate upon these ideas to produce the great creations he produced? To this question, unfortunately, we have to answer, "We do not know." The biography of a specific creation may be more easily approached than that of its creator, despite the many unanswered questions.

II

Stafford's (1991) critical reassessment of the Mozart myths also addresses the question of separating fact from fiction as it relates to Mozart's life, personality, and death. Stafford pays close attention to the evidence for and against assertions, and his focus is on primary evidence, its reliability and its proof. Like Brown, Stafford initially focuses on the myths and legends surrounding Mozart's death.

The vital statistics and dates associated with Mozart's life and death are well known and documented. The major elements of the melodramatic account of his death have been repeatedly reproduced but, as Stafford notes, "most of it is dubious and some of it demonstrably false" (1991, p. 8). Contradictions, questionable authenticity of letters, memoirs, and personal accounts, raise questions. Stafford wonders if Mozart knew he was dying at the end of his life, and "stories of instructing Sussmayr about the Requiem, and rehearsing it on the last day dubious" (Stafford, 1991, pp. 8–9). Many of the eyewitness reports were written years after Mozart's death. They seem to have been embellished and, if not, show the vicissitudes of memory distortions and lapses. That Mozart, a musical genius from childhood, died two months before his thirty-sixth birthday seems accurate. But contradicting reports from supposedly reliable witnesses lead one to question what is true and what is false. Selective publication of edited letters, deliberate falsehoods, contrary accounts from his wife, her second husband, and Mozart's sister and sister-in-law further confound the reader and scholar. Stafford (1991) believes that few new facts remain to be discovered about Mozart's life and death and that most of the reliable evidence is already known. He further believes "that future new work on Mozart's life and death must come from better interpretation of the known evidence" (1991, p. 28).

In discussing Mozart's medical history, Stafford carefully points out the inferences, "the blatant instance of marshalling of evidence to fit a preconceived theory" (p. 70), and these false leads come up with inaccurate conclusions. After examining the various theories about Mozart's fatal illness, Stafford concludes that Mozart's earlier rheumatic fever damaged his heart and that he died of heart failure and infective endocarditis and his damaged heart valves. This diagnosis is the most plausible, least contradicted, although the documents used "to reconstruct Mozart's last days are neither consistent nor entirely trustworthy" (Stafford, 1991, p. 77). Furthermore, Stafford believes Mozart did not work on the *Requiem* on the very day he died. His handwriting was too clear and firm and must have been written at a desk and not in a bed by one who is supposed to have had crippled hands. Constanze apparently lied about several aspects of the *Requiem*'s retrieval by the patron who first commissioned the work. So "gradually a legend crystallized around the Requiem" (Stafford, 1991, p. 79). Constanze and others played a part in fashioning it. It resulted in a romantic aura and thus enhanced the financial value of the work for Constanze. The woven fabric so embroidered made a good story—romantic and fateful. "Mozart's deathbed scene cannot have been noble, tranquil and sentimental. It will have been sordid, characterized by pain and fear" (p. 80).

Reconstruction of past events without complete and reliable data can be wrong. Bias can exist in reconstructing the past. The important element is the biographer, the authenticity of information, and the evidence adduced to support what is being asserted.

Stafford (1991) suggests that the real Mozart is hidden by layers of contradictory myths as is the real Constanze—maligned and treated unjustly, especially by antifeminist stereotypes. More will be said about Constanze's behavior after Mozart's death later in this paper. "Mozart was not a perfect human being, if such a thing is possible. His letters prove that he could be waspish, snobbish, uncharitable and a liar" (p. 140). "No doubt there was exaggeration, but a grain or two of truth must be at bottom of it all. But such a verdict is by no means secure" (p. 141). The history of the legends, carefully tracked, shows how they were plagiarized and perpetuated and how the original source was of doubtful validity. This leaves us with serious open-ended questions that may not be psychologically satisfying or explanatory of his genius, but do not interfere with our appreciation of his creative works.

Stafford (1991) briefly discusses theories that have been offered by psychiatrists and psychoanalysts to explain Mozart's genius. Some have argued that the close relationship with his father was the basis of his inspiration. Others see this relationship as stimulating revolt against the father. Still others see Mozart as compliant and passive submissive or feminine vis-à-vis his father—an inverse oedipal conflict (p. 173). Another suggests he had manic-depressive tendencies. Stafford asks:

> What are such explanations worth? They appear to have scientific credentials, but in fact they are the epitome of the interpretative narrative, which weaves a pattern into the accepted data in the light of a speculative theory. They pick and select the data which accord with their preoccupations. No doubt such narratives on occasion brilliantly reveal a hidden truth; the difficulty is how to test and validate them [1991, p. 174].

This is especially true of someone long dead and where complete facts are unavailable, lending to conjecture, and where evidence may be treated uncritically. Alternative possibilities are not addressed and simple reductionistic explanations are offered for exceedingly complex phenomena and behavior.

Stafford (1991) presents the idea that "Mozart was ready for death, he sensed its imminence, and may have longed for it. The beginnings of this mood can already be found in the last letter he wrote to his dying father in April 1787:

> As death, when we come to consider it closely, is the true goal of our existence, I have formed during the last few years such close relations with this best and truest friend of mankind, that his image is not only no longer terrifying to me, but is indeed very soothing and consoling [Anderson, 1938, p. 907].

Death had recently taken his "dearest and most beloved friend," Count von Hatzfeld, who was in his early thirties. Then in September of the same year, Mozart's physician and friend, Sigmund Barisiri, died at age 29. "The experiences of this year caused a reorientation of his mood; from now on, death was never far from his mind, and the thought of it . . . was perhaps not unwelcome. His presentiment of death finds expression in the spine-tingling music of the stone guest in Don Giovanni" (Stafford, 1991, p. 209). In December 1790, he said goodbye to his friend Haydn who was leaving for London. With tears in his eyes, he said, "I fear . . . that this is the last time we shall see each other" (p. 210). His exhaustion was in evidence, he composed little in 1790, and when he died in 1791, apart from the unfinished *Requiem*, he seemingly left nothing else that was close to completion.

As Stafford (1991) has commented, "There is no indisputable evidence for the hypothesis that Mozart was expecting and half-longing for death in his last years" (p. 220). The last letter to his father may have been an expression of his feelings about his on-coming father's death and his own identification with the paternal part of his own personality. We do not know and probably never will have certainty about this state of feeling. Especially since, in 1791, at the time of his death, there apparently were a number of works in progress, aside from the *Requiem*, including another mass. That Mozart was ill, in all probability from rheumatic fever with cardiac complications, seems likely. If this was so, the chronic heart failure without adequate management could be weakening and culminate in eventual death. That this could affect his work is plausible, although still conjectural.

There were many tragedies and external traumas in Mozart's life (see "Selected Chronology of Mozart and His Family," pp. 163–164). Four of his children became ill and died. His wife was quite ill, requiring expensive spa cures, and extensive medical and pharmaceutical costs. In a letter of 1789, he expresses fear about her condition, especially her bed-sores which interfere with her sleeping, and his anxiety about possible bone pathology. He fears for her life (Stafford, 1991, p. 231). There were serious economic hardships, although the evidence for this is questionable. Stafford cautions the reader to be "mistrustful of imposed patterns" (1991, p. 248), especially when these are designed to give form and significance in narrative form to a life. If one deals with a seamless succession of events and assumes unitary causal connections in order to present a simple overall pattern of meaning and purpose in the face of conflicting evidence or "data," great caution is the order of the day.

III

Deutsch (1963) has written a brief but meaningful chapter on "Some Fallacies in Mozart Biography." In it he raises some of the methodological issues already noted above: the mixing of fact and fiction,

repetitions of earlier tales that remain unverified, inadequate historical and archival studies, the spreading of errors in order to produce
a saleable story. This has been especially true in the case of Mozart
and his *Requiem*. Friedrich Blume (1963) specifically addresses this
issue in his chapter on "Requiem But No Peace," as does Gärtner
(1986) in his more recent book on Constanze Mozart. The posthumous biography of the *Requiem* is filled with error, lies, controversies—all intertwined with fact. The conflict over the authenticity has
been debated repeatedly since 1825 and, as Blume notes, "it would
never be possible to clear up completely all the doubts and questions
raised by the Requiem" (1963, p. 104). He writes that the problems
about the *Requiem* can be divided into three areas:

1. the authenticity problem in the narrower sense,
2. the instrumentation problem,
3. the dating problem [Blume, 1963, p. 105].

The authenticity problem relates to which parts of the composition
are by Mozart himself, which parts were completed by someone else,
and which parts were composed from Mozart's outlines, sketches, or
completely invented by someone else. The instrumentation problem
again refers to whether Mozart himself or someone else was responsible for what emerged. The dating problem concerns itself with
whether the work was composed in the last part of his short life
and what he died of. None of these problems has been satisfactorily
answered. Gärtner (1986) convincingly presents data of how Constanze manipulated and confabulated aspects of the *Requiem* after
Mozart's death for her own personal advantage. There seemingly
were many copies of the *Requiem* that were sold and published when
there supposedly was only one authentic autograph. Different biographers relying on partial or false information perpetuated the myths
and legends surrounding this world famous musical composition.
From all evidence thus far assembled, Blume (1963) concludes that
the *Requiem* was composed in 1791 and that Sussmayr completed the
composition, but not the instrumentation, from Mozart's sketches and
instructions.

Gärtner's book, first published in Germany in 1986, reiterates
and elaborates on the musical mystery of Mozart's *Requiem* and how
Mozart's widow, Constanze, manipulated tales after his death to her
own advantage. She was 29 when Mozart died; she was left with two
small children; she did not have support from Mozart's family, and

there were debts. Despite these obstacles, she was able to manage affairs in a way that was different from her life before her famous husband's early death.

The story of the *Requiem* began on February 14, 1791, when the 20-year-old Countess Anna von Walsegg-Stuppach died. Her husband, Count Franz von Walsegg, commissioned a famous Viennese sculptor to create a monumental tomb for her and, through an unknown intermediary, he commissioned Mozart to compose a requiem mass—a mass for the dead—for her. Mozart agreed to do this, and to the condition that, once delivered, the mass would be the Count's property and that Mozart would not be identified as the composer, but the Count would let it be known that he himself composed it. The Count had previously engaged in such musical plagiarisms and deceptions. This started the story, the further details of which Gärtner (1986) describes in careful and detailed fashion in his book. Mozart never finished the *Requiem*, and because of many false statements attributed to Constanze, Mozart's friends and students turned away from her. Eventually Sussmayr agreed to complete the composition. The legendary enmity between Mozart and Salieri does not seem to have existed. It may have been promulgated by Constanze.

When Constanze delivered the *Requiem* to Count Welsegg:

> [She] concealed from him that another composer had participated in the work's completion, leaving the count to believe he had acquired a genuine Mozart, [and] . . . she had no scruples about having copies made before the score was delivered and selling them as "Mozart's Swan Song," even though the work clearly had become the count's property [Gärtner, 1986, p. 53].

From then on copies of the *Requiem* surfaced everywhere. The Count made the false claim that the *Requiem* was composed by him and, at the same time, Constanze began to market the *Requiem* to publishers. Sussmayr was unhappy because he was denied credit for contributing to the music, although it was not known what and how much he composed. The Count threatened legal action against Constanze, but there was a settlement of his claims. Constanze kept details of the *Requiem* a secret and so she profitted from her manipulations without being detected. She sought to get the maximum profit from the music Mozart left behind when he died (Gärtner, 1986, p. 77). Publishers accused Constanze of fraud and other illegal business activities. Since there were no copyright laws, she could not be prosecuted. Sussmayr, however, continued to expose Constanze's lies and deceptions even though he himself may have claimed to have had more to do with the *Requiem* than was the actual case. The multiple deceptions surrounding the *Requiem* could have been the basis for a Mozart opera if we really knew the accurate details of the unfolding plot. Many of these may never be known to us.

IV

We cannot decide on many of the details of Mozart's death and his composition of the world famous *Requiem*. There are too many evidential gaps, lapses of memory, lost documents, unrecorded information, distorted eye-witness accounts written long after the events being described, contradictions in some of Mozart's own letters, wish-fulfilling recollections, and alternative versions of the same events. Some of these difficulties can never be overcome (Stafford, 1991, p. 264). We lack accurate information and data to understand events in their context over two hundred years ago. These contextual perspectives are different from contemporary contexts. Thus if we interpret past in terms of present, we may be wrong in our understanding. Myths may be cleared away, but we may not know the basis of Mozart's creativity. We may conjecture explanations but conclusions are not firm. What we can do is enjoy Mozart's music, appreciate his contributions to our enrichment, and try to recognize some of the forces that shaped his person.

SELECTED CHRONOLOGY OF MOZART AND HIS FAMILY*

1. January 27, 1756—Wolfgang A. Mozart born. He was the seventh, and second surviving, child of his parents.
2. 1762–1763—Mozart is ill with "rheumatism of the joints."
3. 1765–1766—Mozart falls ill with typhus of the stomach.
4. November 12–21, 1766—Mozart ill with rheumatism of the joints.
5. 1767—Mozart falls ill with smallpox.

---

*Adapted from Hildesheimer (1977), pp. 375–395.

6. 1774—Mozart has a mild illness for six days.
7. 1778—Mozart briefly ill.
8. July 3, 1778—Death of Mozart's mother in Paris.
9. December 25, 1778—Mozart lives with Constanze's family, the Webers.
10. August 4, 1782—Marriage to Constanze Weber.
11. June 17, 1783—Birth of the first child, Raimund Leopold.
12. August 19, 1783—Death of the first child, Raimund Leopold.
13. August–September, 1784—Mozart ill.
14. September 21, 1784—Birth of Mozart's second child, Carl Thomas.
15. October 18, 1786—Birth of Mozart's third child, Johan Thomas Leopold.
16. November 15, 1786—Death of Mozart's third child, Johan Thomas Leopold.
17. May 28, 1787—Death of Mozart's father, Leopold.
18. December 27, 1787—Mozart's fourth child, Theresa, born.
19. June 29, 1788—Daughter Theresa dies.
20. November 16, 1789—Mozart's fifth child, Anna Maria, born, but dies one hour later.
21. July 26, 1791—Birth of Mozart's sixth child, Franz Xavier Wolfgang.
22. Beginning of October, 1791—Work on *Requiem* (?).
23. November 20, 1791—Mozart ill, takes to bed.
24. December 5, 1791—Mozart dies at one o'clock in the morning.

REFERENCES

Anderson, E. (1938), *The Letters of Mozart and His Family*, 3rd ed. New York: W. W. Norton, 1985.

Blume, F. (1963), Requiem but no peace. In: *The Creative World of Mozart*, ed. P. H. Lang. New York: W. W. Norton, 1991, pp. 103–126.

Brown, A. P. (1992), Amadeus and Mozart—Setting the record straight. *Amer. Scholar*, 61:49–66.

Deutsch, O. E. (1963), Some fallacies in Mozart biography. In: *The Creative World of Mozart*, ed. P. H. Lang. New York: W. W. Norton, 1991, pp. 144–149.

Gärtner, H. (1986), *Constanze Mozart—After the Requiem*, trans. R. G. Pauly. Portland, OR: Amadeus Press, 1991.

Hildesheimer, W. (1977), *Mozart*, trans. M. Faber. New York: Vintage Books, 1983.

Stafford, W. (1991), *The Mozart Myths—A Critical Reassessment*. Stanford, CA: Stanford University Press.

13

Genius, Madness, and Health: Examples from Psychobiography

Peter Ostwald, M.D.

Is genius related to madness? Can abnormal mental states be conducive to creative achievement or do they interfere with it? Do geniuses somehow have to suffer because they are eccentric, literally outside the center or the norm?

Such tantalizing questions always recur in discussions about greatly creative, puzzling personalities of the past or present. The "mad genius" notion keeps popping up: One reads and hears about it in popular entertainment and in scientific circles as well: the search for a possible link, a genetic link, a developmental link, a psychodynamic link, a sociocultural link, any kind of linkage between creativity and madness.

Among great composers only Bach seems immune from psychiatric speculation. The earliest biographies of Mozart already suggest that there may have been something unhealthy about his creativity. As the German writer Ludwig Tieck put it in 1812, "if we are obliged to call Mozart insane, then Beethoven cannot be distinguished from the raving mad" (Rosen, 1991). In his chapter in this volume, but much more extensively in his book on Mozart, Dr. Peter Davies alludes to the composer's cyclothymic disorder (Davies, 1989). We also hear about Mozart's "excessive" drinking, a matter of dispute (see Pollock, chapter 12). Earlier, Dr. Gary Gelber gave us some good examples of Mozart's silly clowning, perhaps symptomatic of hypomanic behavior (Gelber, chapter 5).

Instead of attempting to establish links between illness and the unusually high levels of creativity called genius, the opposite point of view sees creativity as essentially a very healthy process, and genius as epitomizing the highest and the best functions of mind and body. Confidence in creative activity is also expressed in the literature on child development, which shows that when imagination, play, and originality are encouraged early in life, the personality becomes both more stable and more flexible (Singer and Singer, 1990).

I tend toward the view of genius as healthy, not only on the basis of clinical experience with gifted musicians (Ostwald, 1992), but also from acquaintance with highly productive people in the arts and sciences, many of whom are exceptionally healthy.

A well-known composer, Kirke Mechem, who has just turned 70 and is in excellent health, told me, "what it's all about is that the creative person must have two ingredients in good balance: imagination and criticism. There are lots and lots of people in this world who are very imaginative," he said. "And there are also a great many people who are highly critical. But you can't get anywhere unless the two qualities are combined. Imagination alone leads to unreal expectations, chaos, and psychosis, while unbridled criticism results in a futile, empty, destructive attitude. It's the constant give-and-take between the two that seems to be the magic."

Artists are generally happiest and at their peak while doing their creative work. Mozart is a perfect example of an artist who felt at his best while making music, both as performer and composer, and would be morose and unhappy if this activity were blocked. Artistic work may be accompanied by a great deal of tension, worry, and sleepless nights, even by anxiety in the clinical sense as well as depression, especially when the creative process is being frustrated for one reason or another. But the incidence of true madness or psychosis seems to be no higher among artists, scientists, or other exceptional people, than in the population at large (Lange-Eichbaum and Kurth, 1967).

HISTORICAL VIEWS ON GENIUS AND MADNESS

Looking at the "mad genius" notion from a historical vantage point, it appears that there have been fluctuating shifts in emphasis, from the one extreme of seeing genius as clearly linked to madness to regarding genius as a healthy phenomenon. By definition genius implies the exceptional, the aberrant, the superhuman, so it is difficult to place such individuals within parameters designed for measuring degrees of health among "ordinary" people. The ancient view placed genius next to godliness, often as a divine personification of masculine creative power. Women were not supposed to have any genius: They had their own goddess, Juno, the sister and also the wife of Jupiter, the "protectress" of women. All power came from the gods: the power to generate life, to wage war, to create beauty, and to destroy. The gods also had the power to drive people mad—to make them go "out of their minds." The Greeks clearly saw links between madness and the extraordinary behavior of great leaders, artists, and philosophers. Plato wrote about the power of genius as "divine madness." Seneca, quoting Aristotle, said "there is no genius without a touch of dementia."

Speculation was rife about the physiological location of exceptional talent, as related to changes in the "humors" of the body. The Renaissance witnessed a revival of the ancient idea that genius was symptomatic of a disturbed bodily state, most likely the product of melancholia caused by the excessive circulation of black bile. Albrecht Dürer, a great artist who suffered from recurring depressive episodes, pictured himself as deeply dejected and surrounded by symbols of decay in a famous etching entitled "Melancholia." The Age of Enlightenment, of which Mozart was a product, turned this theory upside down and envisioned genius as the expression of a supremely well-functioning mind, exhibiting the highest capacities for memory, judgment, and reasoning. The Jewish scholar Moses Mendelssohn, himself a genius from a small town ghetto who translated the Bible into acceptable German and became a court advisor to Frederick the Great, described genius as "a state of perfection of all mental powers working in harmony" (Becker, 1978, p. 25).

After that period of enlightenment came revolutions and all the outpouring of passion called Romanticism. It was the era of storm and stress—*Sturm und Drang*—as Goethe called it, and the period during the nineteenth century especially, which generated with great energy what sociologist George Becker (1978) terms "the Mad Genius Controversy." That was stimulated by the introspective accounts of many artists and poets of the Romantic Era who wrote about themselves as suffering a great deal, being mentally disturbed and extremely moody, and by the nineteenth-century physicians and scientists who promoted the concept of "degeneration."

THE INFLUENCE OF ARTISTS

In letters and diaries, artists have commented extensively and intro-spectively on their emotional ups and downs and tried in various ways to symbolize mood swings in their artistic productions. Ludwig van Beethoven, for example, actually gave the title "La Malinconia" to the last movement of his String Quartet opus 18, number 6, showing in musical terms what it felt like to fluctuate back and forth from a subdued, inhibited, quiet mood (the opening and recurring Adagio), to one which was jumpy, jolly, and exuberant (the intervening Alle-gro). That does not make for a diagnosis of manic–depressive disor-der—clinical evidence for this disease would have to be submit-ted—but it does show the composer's conscious awareness of the effect upon his composition of changing levels of emotional tension. In a later work, his String Quartet opus 132, Beethoven went a step fur-ther, writing above the slow movement that it was a song of thanks to express his gratitude for having recovered from a serious illness.

Composer Robert Schumann repeatedly described himself as go-ing mad and fulfilled this self-prophecy by entering a psychiatric hospital two years before his suicide. More than anyone in the field of music, he epitomizes the "mad genius" struggle (Ostwald, 1985). During adolescence, Schumann became aware of various "noises" and "voices" in his head, usually following bouts of heavy drinking or other intoxicating experiences. The voices inspired him to write music and poetry, while the noises distracted and depressed him. He often experienced a split in his personality, which he described as alternat-ing between a subdued, pensive, sensitive, introverted, feminine char-acter called "Eusebius" (after an early Christian martyr) and an ag-gressive, violent, quixotic, and masculine character called "Florestan" (after the hero of Beethoven's opera *Fidelio*). The extreme symbol of the duality experienced by creative people in the nineteenth century is, of course, Stevenson's *The Strange Case of Dr. Jekyll and Mr. Hyde* (1886).

THE INFLUENCE OF SCIENTISTS

During the nineteenth century, progress was made in explaining the causes of serious illnesses such as epilepsy, syphilis, and tuberculosis, whose victims included some of the great geniuses: Chopin, who died of tuberculosis; van Gogh, who was probably epileptic (or, according to a more recent theory, had a metabolic disorder causing sensorimotor crises), and Franz Schubert, who contracted syphilis, most probably from a homosexual prostitute.

These artists continue to be highly visible and arouse more curiosity and stimulate more controversy than does the "average" patient. It was Jean-Jacques Moreau (1859), in France, who first proposed the degeneration theory to explain various medical diseases rampant in the nineteenth century and his idea caught on quickly. Degeneration was a physical explanation, based partly on notions about the racial transmission of biologically negative features and partly on the study of pathology, mainly from autopsies, but it had psychological and social implications. The idea of degeneration spread quickly throughout Europe and became the leading scientific concept used by physicians to explain a whole host of problems, including mental deficiency, criminal behavior, psychosis, and genius.

The man who did more than anyone to forge a hypothetical link between genius and madness was the Italian psychiatrist and criminologist Cesare Lombroso, 1836–1909. He was almost a fanatic on the subject and wrote many books which were translated and circulated widely. Let me present just a few quotations from one of Lombroso's books, *The Man of Genius* (first published in 1890), to give a flavor of his thinking: "I discover in genius various characteristics of degeneration which are the foundation of nearly all forms of congenital mental abnormality." He was rather deprecating: "Geniuses are short, emaciated, sterile, microcephalic, stupid, and ugly. . . . lacking in tact, in moderation, in the sense of practical life, in the virtues useful in social affairs" (Lombroso, 1913, p. vii).

Dr. Gelber (chapter 5) told us that Mozart viewed himself as short, pockmarked, and not the most diplomatic person in society. That would have fit Lombroso's stereotype.

These stereotypes of genius quickly became popular. Here's another statement from Lombroso (1913): "That certain great men of genius have been insane permits us to presume the existence of a lesser degree of psychosis in other men of genius" (p. ix). Nowadays we simply wouldn't accept the idea that because certain people are mentally ill, all such people must be somewhat mentally ill too! But Lombroso was a dedicated scientist, intent on proving his thesis; he collected the art of the insane and he collected the brains of both psychotic patients and geniuses. One of his ideas was that geniuses had smaller brains than normal people, and his books contain many such demonstrations. Today we know that brain size per se is no criterion of mental ability, and our neuroscientists have far more sophisticated techniques, such as MRI and PET scanning, to investigate the connections between brain structures and psychological functions.

Lombroso's "discoveries" triggered an avalanche of publications about the supposed connection between genius and neurological degeneration. Some authors agreed that great men had pathological brains. For example, in his famous book *The Insanity of Genius*, the British psychologist J. F. Nisbet (1912) professed the theory that painters have diseased nerve cells in the visual cortex of the brain, while with musicians "the auditory and general motor areas are affected." According to Nisbet:

> Mozart, in the height of his activity, lived in a delirium of invention, often working so hard that, as he himself expressed it, he did not know whether his head was on or off. . . . Wherever he happened to be, Mozart was incessantly preoccupied with musical thoughts. . . . He was always strumming—on his hat, his watch-fob, the table, the chairs, as if he were at the piano, and even in conversation with his friends he seemed to be carrying on an under-train of musical thought. . . . At the opera, his friends could tell by the restless movements of his hands, by his look, and the motion of his lips as if he were singing or whistling, that he was entirely engrossed by his internal musical activity. . . . Other great composers have similarly been controlled by the automatic forces of their brain [Nisbet, 1912, pp. 284–286].

There were also those who disagreed with Lombroso. The German physician W. Hirsch, for example, asserted that the extraordinary accomplishments of a genius like Mozart cannot possibly be attributed to brain degeneration. On the contrary, he wrote, a refinement of specific psychic functions must be involved:

> It is to be presumed that musical talent depends upon a specially refined development of a certain acoustic centre, although its

location at present escapes our knowledge. . . . In his inexhaustible and restlessly working fancy, Mozart was very much like Goethe. His works most commonly lay ready-made in his memory when he began to set them down on paper. . . . Here again is a high refinement of a universal psychical phenomenon. . . . We hardly know which most to admire, his stupendous talent or his creative genius. Mozart's rich fancy, like that of Goethe, was directed by a high intellectual faculty which checked its boilings over, held the ideas to an ordered sequence, and eliminated disturbing elements. Mozart's capacity of concentrating his attention upon what was in his mind, and of shutting out all disturbing perceptions of sense, was tremendous. . . . But wherever it was worth while to pay attention to the outer world, and to take in outward impressions of sense, he had an equally high capacity for that. His fancy received rich aliment from the action of his intellect [Hirsch, 1897, pp. 56–58].

THEORIES ON CREATIVITY AND MADNESS TODAY

As we approach the end of the twentieth century, a swing of opinion toward the idea of mood disorder as contributing significantly to the creative process is becoming apparent. For example, in his 1975 Benjamin Rush Lecture to the American Psychiatric Association, the great literary scholar and biographer Leon Edel emphasized that many creative people experience powerful feelings of sadness, depression, and "benign megalomania." But these are not necessarily pathological states: "I see a particular sadness. We might say it is simply the sadness of life, but it is a sadness that somehow becomes a generating motor, a link in the chain of power that makes the artist persist, even when he has lived an experience, to transform it within his medium. . . . Out of world-sadness, out of tristimania, immortal and durable things are brought into being" (Edel, 1975, pp. 1008, 1012).

In a series of studies of professional writers and their families, psychiatrist Nancy Andreasen (1988) found an unusually high incidence of affective-spectrum disease (depression, bipolar affective disorder, alcoholism, and suicide) suggesting a possible genetic link. Psychologist Kay Jamison is trying to extend this hypothetical relationship between creativity and bipolar disorder to other groups and believes that among famous composers, Handel, Mahler, Berlioz, Schumann, and Hugo Wolf were manic-depressive (Goodwin and

Jamison, 1990). There can be little doubt that Schumann and Wolf were so afflicted. But it seems unlikely that Handel was manic-depressive (Frosch, 1989), and the clinical evidence supporting this diagnosis for Mahler and Berlioz also is weak.

A statistical study of a much larger group of artists by psychiatrist Hagop Akiskal also fails to strengthen the connection between bipolarity and creativity. Akiskal suggests that the "softer" bipolar conditions (i.e., DSM-III-R Bipolar 2 and 3 groups [APA, 1987]) may be related to creativity but that this relationship is not impressive. Only 8 percent of the "soft bipolars" in his caseload were known to be artistic; the remaining 92 percent were not. "There is a group of temperaments related to the affective spectrum which can lead to various outcomes, one of which can be creative," says Akiskal (1991). "Why does this happen? The answer is not easy. Chance? Greater intelligence? Choice? Environment? These factors are obviously important, and it could be that mental illness is the product of a mismatch between artistic temperament and an environment that is non-supportive or inhibiting." A recent book, *The Key to Genius* by D. Jablow Hershman and Julian Lieb, is less cautious in attempting to link creativity with manic-depression.

> [The authors] believe that manic energy cycling with depressive introspection intensifies the creative process and that mania— when harnessed—may simply be what is commonly called "the creative urge." Manic exuberance provides the confidence and defiance of criticism that are indispensable when charting new frontiers, and depression offers the self-examination and pursuit of perfection required to refine inventive works [Crusack, 1991].

Unfortunately this attractive formulation stems from the study of such men as Newton, Beethoven, Dickens, and Van Gogh, whose illnesses cannot be convincingly diagnosed as bipolar affective disorder.

FROM PATHOGRAPHY TO PSYCHOBIOGRAPHY

Where does the raw data about geniuses come from? What enables physicians, psychologists, and other scholars writing about people like Mozart to form theories regarding their personalities and mental development? One way, of course, is through biographical research, digging out the facts about geniuses accumulated in the course of time by those who are inclined and trained to study human lives. The art of biography is an ancient one, practiced at first by those who wanted to idolize or to denigrate historical figures. Gradually, biography evolved into a more objective pursuit, aiming to examine individual achievements and failures in a historical context. Toward the end of the nineteenth century and under the influence of Romanticism and the theories of degeneration mentioned above, biography veered briefly in the direction of *pathography*, a term coined by the Leipzig neurologist Paul Moebius, who wrote books about Goethe, Schumann, and other unusually gifted people (Schiller, 1982). These were extensive case histories that sought to find evidence for disease states that might be related to their creative behavior. For example, Moebius (1906) thought that changes in Robert Schumann's compositional style could be attributed to the effects of a schizophrenic process.

Moebius's work was known to Sigmund Freud, who also began his career as a neurologist. But Freud, after working with Charcot, Breuer, and other physicians interested in using hypnosis to treat hysteria, formulated theories about the mind which moved radically away from organic explanations based on brain pathology to psychological processes. In postulating a dynamic unconscious that contained not only instinctual motivations but also repressed memories of childhood events, Freud changed the face of psychiatry. In addition to extensive case reports about patients he had psychoanalyzed, Freud wrote essays about people he could not have examined or treated: Leonardo da Vinci, Michelangelo, Dostoevsky, for example. His aim was to delineate the effects of infantile sexuality, the Oedipus complex, and other unconscious determinants of symbolic behavior not only in people who could be called neurotic, but also among the artistic and creative.

Central to Freud's theory of creativity was the concept of "sublimation," a defense mechanism that allowed the ego to transform unacceptable libidinal and aggressive tendencies into socially desirable acts. Creativeness could now be seen as the obverse of destructiveness: How the two tendencies interacted and at what point to label a specific piece of behavior pathological became problems for social science as well as psychiatry.

It remained for Erik Erikson, a nonmedical psychoanalyst, to broaden the field to include cultural, historical, and social factors in describing exceptional lives. Erikson's books, especially his monumental studies of Martin Luther and Mohandas K. Gandhi, set the stage for psychobiography, explorations based on awareness of psychological principles, including the effects of unconscious motivation and transference on the part of the biographer (Runyan, 1982).

PSYCHOBIOGRAPHIES OF MUSICIANS

One of the first musicians to have been a subject for psychobiographical investigation was Gustav Mahler, the prodigiously talented and ambitious pianist, conductor, and composer. During a marital crisis in 1910, Mahler had actually sought consultation with Freud. As the minutes of the Vienna Psychoanalytic Society show (Ostwald, 1991b), Freud was reluctant to discuss details of the Mahler case with his colleagues, but many years after the composer's death he did reveal certain crucial facts, first to Marie Bonaparte and then to Theodore Reik. According to Freud, Mahler had a strong fixation on his mother which led to sexual inhibitions and he had been traumatized during childhood by his father. Reik incorporated aspects of Mahler's life into his book *The Haunting Melody* (1953), a free-associative autobiography that describes music as a language especially suited to the elaboration of unconscious thoughts. Later psychobiographical studies of Mahler have focused on his reactions to repeated sibling loss (Pollock, 1990) and physical disease (Feder, 1978), and his heroic efforts to achieve inner stability through musical composition, much of it devoted to themes of mourning and resurrection.

Ludwig van Beethoven has long been of interest to biographers. A psychoanalytic study by Sterba and Sterba (1954), of Beethoven's relationship with his nephew whom he adopted as a son, created considerable controversy, in part because of the emphasis on homosexual dynamics in their ill-fated relationship. A more comprehensive psychobiography of the composer appeared in 1977 in which Maynard Solomon explored factors motivating both Beethoven's extraordinary creativity and his severely handicapped personality: a delusional sense of his paternity, conflicts between self-isolation and yearning for love, and the hazards of deafness and other physical diseases (Solomon, 1977).

More recently Solomon (1989) tackled the problem of Franz Schubert's homosexuality, and he has worked on aspects of Mozart's career in preparation for a full-scale psychobiography. A concluding remark from Solomon's paper about Mozart's Zoroastrian riddles is pertinent to our thesis about the essential difference between creative genius and psychotic madness: "In his work, the artist finds ways symbolically to repair psychic injuries and object losses, to neutralize anxieties. But he does this by means of socially developed techniques and forms of art, so that what had been private and opaque becomes a shared communication" (Solomon, 1990, p. 420).

Robert Schumann also demonstrated this capacity for transforming disturbing aspects of the self into artistic products. He discovered that while practicing and improvising at the piano it was possible not only to reduce his inner distress but also to capture certain of his mood states in musical compositions (Ostwald, 1985). After an episode of acute, disorganizing, suicidal panic when he was in his early twenties, caused in part by physical problems with his right hand that threatened to curtail his career as a virtuoso, Schumann became a music critic. This allowed him to sublimate aggressive and destructive impulses into literary work, for the benefit of other musicians who gained attention through Schumann's writings, while at the same time he could publicly proclaim his own views on romanticism in music. Schumann's maturation as a composer coincided with his relationship and marriage to the pianist Clara Wieck; despite repeated depressive illnesses he worked productively until his midforties, when hospitalization became necessary after a catastrophically disruptive psychotic episode. Tragically, his enforced isolation in an asylum, his loss of contact with his wife and children, as well as the lack of specific treatment and perhaps some irremedial organic changes, put a stop to Schumann's creativity.

CONVERGENCE BETWEEN ILLNESS AND CREATIVITY

Schumann's life is but one example of the coexistence within a single individual of successful creative tendencies along with disruptive states of mental disorder. It raises again our initial question: whether creativity and psychosis have something in common. This question is important to our theoretical understanding of creativity. It also arises whenever gifted but disturbed people inquire about psychiatric care and anxiously want to know if the quality or quantity of their creative output will be affected by treatment.

Albert Rothenberg, a psychoanalyst with a long-standing interest in this problem, sought to address these issues by debunking some of the "old myths" about creativity. As Rothenberg (1990) points out, creativity does not arise from divine inspiration, does not simply well up from the unconscious, and is not a "miraculous faculty" or the product of superior intelligence. What creative people have in common is that they use special "translogical" modes of thinking while creating. There is nothing pathological about these patterns of thinking, nor do they arise from pathological motivations. On the contrary, their roots are highly adaptive and healthy. There seems to be no specific personality type or style associated with outstanding creativity. On standard IQ tests, creative people do not always test as exceptionally intelligent. Only one characteristic—motivation—is present in all creative people and seems related to a particular family situation: Almost always there is one parent who tried some field of creativity but was not hugely successful. "The creative person . . . strives to fulfill a parent's implicit, unrealized yearnings" (Rothenberg, 1990, p. 13).

Two modes of translogical thinking have been identified. The first is called "janusian" thinking, a term derived from the Roman deity Janus, guardian of the temple gates, whose face looked forward and backward at the same time. Creativity is characterized by this janusian process, whereby it is possible to think simultaneously of multiple opposites or antitheses. Freud had described the occurrence of opposites or contradictions in thought as part of the primary process characteristic of childhood, dreaming, neurosis, and other unconscious functions; the Vienna-born philosopher Ludwig Wittgenstein commented on it as well (Monk, 1990). Rothenberg's point is that the creative person not only formulates simultaneities and antitheses *consciously* but develops these formulations into integrated and well-organized entities—original works of art, music, writing, inventions, or scientific discoveries. Psychotics, by contrast, seem unaware of the contradictions and antitheses in their thinking; they become delusional, self-defeating, or destructive.

The second mode of translogical thinking identified by Rothenberg is called the "homospatial" process. Here two or more separate objects are conceived as occupying the same space at the same time. Such sensoricognitive experiences can be overwhelming and disorganizing for a psychotic person. But the creative process benefits from homospatiality: fleeting sensory impressions of a contradictory nature can lead to the articulation of new identities and the construction of metaphors. In art, foreground and background are brought into a single plane; in music, signal and noise are brought into harmony; in literature, overlapping entities are synthesized into poetic imagery. Thus, while janusian and homospatial processes are common to both psychosis and creativity, Rothenberg sees them as fulfilling different purposes. "Artworks are communications in a sense that psychological symptoms never are or can be. . . . Although creative people may be psychotic at various periods in their lives . . . they cannot be psychotic at the same time they are engaged in a creative process, or it will not be successful. Homospatial and janusian processes are healthy ones" (Rothenberg, 1990, pp. 46, 36).

In his stimulating book *Creative Malady*, the British physician and Nobel laureate Sir George Pickering (1974) adopted an alternative approach, suggesting that by forcing patients to change their life style, turn inwards, and seek more leisure for their work, disease may exert a beneficial influence on the creative process. His case examples include Marcel Proust, confined by asthma to his cork-lined room, where he created his literary masterpiece in bed; Sigmund Freud, whose obsessional neurosis catalyzed experiments with free association leading to psychoanalysis; Charles Darwin, forced by invalidism to retreat from society and work on the theory of evolution; Florence Nightingale, who turned private suffering into a compassionate nursing career; Mary Baker Eddy, whose physical frailty and neurotic suffering led her to the principles of Christian Science, and Elizabeth Barrett Browning, whose impaired health fostered achievement as a poet.

Other stresses besides poor health generate creativity. Psychoanalyst George Pollock has been particularly eloquent in elucidating the role of bereavement in stimulating this process. His studies of Gustav Mahler, Käthe Kollwitz, Charles Chaplin, and other unusually productive and successful individuals show very clearly how the loss of parents or siblings, especially early in life, not only induces a pattern of reparative behavior but enforces certain "thematic perseverations" in the creative activity (Pollock, 1978). For example, at age 14 the painter René Magritte viewed his mother's corpse after she drowned herself, an event that evidently led him to question the meaning of human existence. While leading an outwardly conventional and conservative life, through his art and especially his self-portraits Magritte revealed an almost obsessional concern with ambivalent symbols, many of them in a humorous context. Memories of his adolescent trauma often appear in Magritte's paintings, where mermaids and curiously dismembered women serve as disguised flashbacks to the shattering vision of his drowned mother.

The topic of "psychotic art," or how people who are deeply disturbed express themselves artistically (MacGregor, 1989) cannot be addressed here in detail. Instead, I would like to turn to a case presentation, the dancer Vaslav Nijinsky who, like Mozart, ascended to fame early in life but after he was 30 saw his brilliant career collapse.

A CASE STUDY OF GENIUS AND MADNESS

Unlike Mozart, who died at age 35, Nijinsky (1889–1950) lived to be 61, but the last half of his life was spent as a psychiatric invalid (Ostwald, 1991a). I present this case here for two reasons: first, to review what was brought out earlier in this volume by David Henry Feldman about the ten criteria that appear necessary in the evolution of child prodigy to genius, and second, to suggest that the same criteria might also apply when one examines the devolution from genius to madness. The ten criteria given by Feldman (chapter 2) are:

Family history
First-born (or surviving) male
Specific talents
Sufficient resources
Single-mindedness
Inner confidence
Arouses ambivalence
Developmental crisis
Ten years to develop a unique style
Childlike qualities as an adult

FAMILY HISTORY

Both of Vaslav Nijinsky's parents were dancers. Thus an inclination for him to be involved in artistic expression through body movement was embedded in the boy's family. His mother had been performing

in ballet since her own childhood; his father was a strikingly handsome and athletic dancer, famous for his unusually high leaps and
his dramatic talent. Both worked in various theaters, circuses, and
opera houses throughout their homeland, Poland, and in Russia
where Vaslav was born. He studied with his father and strongly identified with him. But it was an insecure childhood, with much hectic
traveling, financial insecurity, and instability in the parents' relationship to each other as well as to their children. The mother was often
depressed, and the father, five years her junior, had an explosive
personality style. He abused his wife and children, and abandoned
them when Vaslav was 8 years old, a loss to which the boy responded
with depression and self-isolation, followed by a tendency toward
excessive dependency on older men. Clearly, Nijinsky's family history
was conducive to both artistic achievement and psychopathology.

First-Born (or Surviving) Male

Vaslav was the second of three children, all of them pressed into
dancing at an early age. However, the oldest child, Stanislav, had
become disabled as a result of a head injury sustained when as an
infant he fell out of a window (possible evidence of child neglect). His
intellectual and emotional impairment became more troublesome as
the boy approached adolescence, when he was placed in a state institution for the rest of his life. This tragedy not only put Vaslav in position
as the surviving son, capturing and holding the spotlight as a child
prodigy dancer, but instilled in him both curiosity and dread regarding mental disease. Visits to his crippled brother in the hospital were
disturbing and may have stimulated Nijinsky's lifelong interest in
pathological postures and movements observed among neuropsychiatric patients. As a dancer and choreographer he incorporated highly
unorthodox and sometimes shocking movements into his ballets.
After becoming a psychiatric patient himself, he often adopted strikingly bizarre postures. Through all of this, his younger sister Bronis-
lava, much like Mozart's older sister Nannerl, had a stabilizing influence on the family; following Vaslav's decline she carried on their
tradition of balletic originality.

SPECIFIC TALENTS

The word *talent* implies innate abilities that propel certain individuals to go much further than their relatively ungifted peers in pursuing a career. Howard Gardner (1983) uses the term *special intelligence* and identifies at least seven "domains" of behavior for which certain youngsters seem especially gifted or "pretuned"—mathematics, abstract reasoning, music, athletics, verbal skills, spatial relationships, and dealing with people. Nijinsky clearly was most talented in body movement relying on athletic, musical, and kinesthetic abilities. He was much weaker in the verbal–intellectual sphere of literary, rational, and interpersonal skills. He specialized in using his face and body to portray the entire range of human emotion, from abject sadness through sensitive affection, puzzlement, delight, humor, and erotic excitement, to frenzy and violence in roles that electrified audiences, such as Harlequin in *Carnaval*; the puppet in *Petrushka*; the Golden Slave in *Scheherazade*; the Faun in *L'Apres-midi d'un Faune*, and many other unforgettable characters. Nijinsky also had a phenomenal talent for leaping: As a child he modeled it after his father and subsequently honed it through constant practice to give the illusion of being suspended in space. "It's simple," he is supposed to have said, "all you have to do is go up and then stay there for a while."

Nijinsky's particular talents led to complications after he was hospitalized. Excellence in facial mimicry made it difficult for his psychiatrists to arrive at a fitting diagnosis, as the dancer would portray various states of psychosis he had observed in his brother and other patients. Even experts like Eugen Bleuler and Ludwig Binswanger were confused: Was Nijinsky catatonic, or was he play acting? And his extraordinary leaps made him dangerous on the wards where he would suddenly take off and land on someone, once nearly choking an attendant to death. For many years Nijinsky abandoned speech altogether. Thus we see his great talent for nonverbal communication serving first artistic then psychopathological ends.

SUFFICIENT RESOURCES

His mother had obtained for him the best training in classical ballet then available, a scholarship at the Imperial Ballet School of St. Petersburg. Despite his academic deficiencies Nijinsky graduated at age 18 with great distinction, and a guarantee of lifetime employment in Russia's Imperial Theaters, plus an adequate retirement pension which for ballet dancers usually began in the fourth or fifth decade of life. Regimentation was extreme in this environment. The white-washed school dormitories, with rows of identical white beds, resembled hospital wards. The students wore uniforms. Their social behavior was rigidly controlled, and fraternizing with the opposite sex was forbidden. Nijinsky became very dependent on this system. Following his graduation he complained: "I did not know how to dress. I was used to uniforms. I did not like civilian dress and therefore did not know how to wear it. . . . I felt free but the freedom terrified me. . . . I did not know life" (Nijinsky, 1913, pp. 92–93). This helpless dependency became a lifelong trait. When he joined the Ballets Russes, all his basic needs were met by his lover and mentor, Sergei Diaghilev, who provided lodging, meals, clothing, recreation, and supervised a heavy daily work schedule. Nijinsky never learned how to manage his own affairs.

SINGLE-MINDEDNESS

Nijinsky had but a single purpose in life: to perfect his body as an instrument of supreme artistic appeal. Exercise gave him optimal muscularity, coordination, and grace. For hours and days he would meditate, fantasize, and practice new character roles. This total absorption in make-believe assured Nijinsky's excellence as a dancer and contributed to his enormous success. But it also left him without practical knowledge of things outside the theater world, and probably accentuated his social awkwardness. He was a maladroit conversationalist, making odd quixotic remarks or withdrawing into stony silence. One admirer, Misia Sert, called him an "idiot of genius." While on stage, he was totally absorbed in creating a character, so convincingly that audiences felt he literally *was* Petrushka, the Spectre de la Rose, or some other fantastic creature. Offstage, despite his short stature and unprepossessing physical appearance, he radiated a mysterious sexual attractiveness. Later, when he became a psychiatric patient, Nijinsky's single-mindedness kept him ensnared in psychotic delusions. He believed himself to be God, and felt in mortal danger of being killed. He retreated into catatonic stupors, interrupted by frenzied spells of maniacal destructiveness.

INNER CONFIDENCE

Nijinsky's inner confidence was manifest in unremitting willfulness at pushing his own ideas forward despite resistance. As a dancer in his teens he had stretched the rules of classical ballet to the limit, imposing fresh interpretations upon each role he was asked to dance, injecting highly original and often very difficult variations into the standard ballet repertoire. As a member of the Diaghilev company he was invited to create entirely new roles and did so with enormous flair and cockiness. As a choreographer he confidently broke the traditional barriers of dance symbolism by fashioning movements that were extremely innovative but often considered ugly and unphysiological. In the throes of his psychosis he would convincingly dance roles that reflected his religious delusions and paranoid fantasies.

AROUSES AMBIVALENCE

Nijinsky's dancing stirred great enthusiasm as well as enormous resistance. As a prodigious young artist he was quickly elevated to the status of a superstar and dubbed "God of the Dance," flattery that might have contributed to his later, delusional equation of self with God. But along the way he was also ruthlessly criticized for dancing in ways that seemed obscene, bestial, disgusting, or effeminate. One critic denigrated Nijinsky's "Faune" as "incontinent, with vile movements of erotic bestiality and gestures of heavy shamelessness," while sculptor Auguste Rodin (at Diaghilev's request) praised him as "the ideal model, whom one longs to draw and sculpt" (Ostwald, 1991a, p. 60). Despite their admiration for Nijinsky, few of his contemporaries seemed able to understand what he was trying to express and it is only today, forty years after his death, that through conscientious reconstructions his visionary ballets are being seen widely and are receiving the admiration they deserve.

DEVELOPMENTAL CRISIS

Mozart's developmental crisis occurred during his twenty-sixth year, after his long-considered decision to separate from his father, move to Vienna, and get married, steps which greatly benefitted his career and were to lead to his most mature compositions (Braunbehrens, 1990). An analogous crisis in Nijinsky's life at age 24 destabilized his career and had disastrous effects on his creativity. While separated from Diaghilev during a tour of South America, Nijinsky impulsively decided to marry Romola Pulszky, a flirtatious young woman who had been following him around for many months. She sought to control and manipulate Nijinsky much as Diaghilev had done, but lacked his vision and artistic resources. Dismissed from the Ballets Russes by the jealous Diaghilev, Nijinsky tried and failed to form a ballet company of his own with his sister. With no other opportunity to dance in public, the charismatic Nijinsky panicked and became depressed, developed somatic symptoms, and was diagnosed by doctors in London, Vienna, and Budapest as suffering from "neurasthenia," a diagnosis he had also received three years earlier from a physician in Russia. During his marriage, Nijinsky fathered two children but adapted poorly to family life. After age 30 he became psychotically disturbed.

It is debatable whether one should attempt to normalize a genius. Constanze Mozart has been blamed, unfairly perhaps, for allegedly failing to appreciate her husband's greatness and not giving him enough emotional support. Romola Nijinsky, too, has been held responsible for her husband's problems. She could not accept his sexual nonconformity, which ranged from homosexuality with older men, through self-absorbed masturbation, to flagrant promiscuity with female prostitutes. (But Romola, after her husband became psychotic, herself engaged exclusively in lesbian relationships.) She tended alternately to dominate and to abandon him. The ambivalence in their relationship proved so overwhelming that separation preliminary to divorce was finally recommended in 1919 when Eugen Bleuler saw the couple in psychiatric consultation. By then, however, the dancer, now 30 and beginning to lose his physical attractiveness, had become so erratic, unpredictable, and hostile that hospitalization seemed indicated, an unfitting resolution of his developmental crisis.

TEN YEARS TO DEVELOP HIS UNIQUE STYLE

Mozart died after ten years of fabulous productivity and stupendous artistic growth, following his developmental crisis at age 25. Nijinsky also had a decade in which to exploit fully his potential as a creative dancer and choreographer. His last and most original ballet *Till Eulenspiegel,* had been mounted in 1916 when he was rehired by Diaghilev to appear with the Ballets Russes on a tour of the United States. After that, Nijinsky thought of returning to Russia, where he hoped to lead a nomadic existence, the life of a simple peasant. Blocked by depressive episodes and the lack of opportunity for producing ballets in Switzerland, he began confining his efforts to obsessive drawing of circles, mandalalike patterns varying from originality to stereotypy.

CHILDLIKE QUALITIES AS AN ADULT

The negative side of Nijinsky's personality was characterized by naïveté, gullibility, and helplessness, which as he grew older and more chronically psychotic overbalanced the positive side, his gracefulness, charm, immense kinesthetic skill, and originality. Always handicapped in verbal communication, he grew silent, sullen, silly, menacing, coarse, and incontinent. He gave up all civilized habits, threw his food, jumped around like an animal, masturbated openly, and sometimes attacked others. At first he pretended that all this regressive behavior was designed to make him look like a "lunatic," a replica of his dead psychotic brother. "People like eccentrics and they will therfore leave me alone, saying that I am a 'mad clown' " he wrote in a notebook (Ostwald, 1991a, p. 178). His first psychotherapist, the well-known psychoanalyst Ludwig Binswanger, described many scenes in the hospital where Nijinsky would try to enact the role of a madman and impress the staff and other patients with his complete mastery of illness. "The impression he makes, and the complete art of his pantomime, is most thoroughly studied and 'truthful' " (Ostwald, 1991a, p. 217). But as the years rolled by, Nijinsky's behavior became more devoid of thoughtful planning. Occasionally there were brief, miraculous periods of lucidity when he would speak, experience pleasure, and dance again, but only when unusual events prompted this behavior; for instance at the end of World War II when Russian troops entered the area where he was staying and urged him to join their singing and dancing, or in England, after the war when he mingled with dancers from the Paris Opera.

Just before he died in 1950, like Mozart in 1791, from renal failure, Nijinsky engaged in dancelike movements with his arms, smiled in a childlike way, and, according to Romola, asked for his mother. Thus the circle was completed: birth into a dancing family, child prodigy dancer, world ballet superstar, innovative choreographer, ten years of creative genius, thirty years of psychotic inactivity and destructive madness, then death.

CONCLUSION

Activity that leads to the production of something new, useful, and of lasting value for society can hardly be considered pathological. Yet the idea persists that highly creative people, especially outstanding "geniuses," have been disease-prone or vulnerable to madness. Genius is indeed a very rare phenomenon. One of the most conscientious researchers, the German psychiatrist Wilhelm Lange-Eichbaum, counted fewer than 600 geniuses since the beginning of recorded history (Lange-Eichbaum and Kurth, 1967). These are such unique individuals that it is difficult to make generalizations about their personalities, psychopathology, or health status.

A historical review has been given to show shifting attitudes regarding this problem. Psychobiographical research underscores the vast difference between creativity, which is fundamentally productive, and madness, which is destructive.

A necessary condition for creative work is that gifted individuals be provided with training, tools, and opportunities. In addition, it seems that unhappiness, conflict, stress, or even illness may at times enhance a creative tendency, the striving to seek new meanings and modify reality in ways that are socially useful. There is no guarantee, of course, that such visions and changes will please everyone or be generally accepted. The highly creative person risks being misunderstood, rejected, and even negatively labeled as an eccentric or madman. On the other hand, when society is moved by creative individuals and their products, recognizes their value, uses and enjoys them, there often follows an accumulation of respect and fame for these people, ultimately even attribution to them of the term *genius*.

Highly creative people often are or feel themselves to be out of step with their social environment, and attempts to normalize them tend to be resisted. They have the capacity greatly to enhance the lives of others and to enrich their culture. Adulation or neglect can affect their social behavior. When their work is thwarted by external or internal impediments, the risk to them of disease may be heightened. Parents, teachers, physicians, and others in positions of authority have the responsibility to understand the creative process and to protect and encourage creativity in healthy people and in sick people (Ostwald, 1992).

REFERENCES

Akiskal, H. (1991), Discussion of creativity and depression. Paper presented at the Annual Meeting of the Northern California Psychiatric Society, Berkeley, California.

American Psychiatric Association (1987), *Diagnostic and Statistical Manual of Mental Disorders*, 3rd ed. rev. (DSM-III-R). Washington, DC: American Psychiatric Press.

Andreasen, N. C. (1988), Creativity and mental illness: Prevalence rates in writers and their first-degree relatives. *Amer. J. Psychiatry*, 144:1288–1292.

Becker, G. (1978), *The Mad Genius Controversy: A Study in the Sociology of Deviance*. Beverly Hills, CA: Sage.

Braunbehrens, V. (1990), *Mozart in Vienna, 1781–1791*, trans. T. Bell. New York: Grove Weidenfeld.

Crusack, J. R. (1991), Review of *The Key to Genius* by D. J. Hershman and Julian Lieb. *Amer. J. Psychiatry*, 142:1747–1748.

Davies, P. (1989), *Mozart in Person: His Character and Health*. Westport, CT: Greenwood.

Edel, L. (1975), The madness of art. *Amer. J. Psychiatry*, 132:1005–1012.

Feder, S. (1978), Gustav Mahler, dying. *Internat. J. Psycho-Anal.*, 5:125–148.

Frosch, W. (1989), The "case" of George Frideric Handel. *N. Eng. J. Med.*, 321:765–769.

Gardner, H. (1983), *Frames of Mind: The Theory of Multiple Intelligences*. New York: Basic Books.

Goodwin, F. C., & Jamison, K. R. (1990), *Manic-Depressive Illness*. New York: Oxford University Press.

Hershman, D. J., & Lieb, J. (1988), *The Key to Genius*. Buffalo, NY: Prometheus Books.

Hirsch, W. (1897), *Genius and Degeneration: A Psychological Study*. London: Hienemann.

Kirstein, L. (1975), *Nijinsky Dancing*. New York: Alfred A. Knopf.

Lange-Eichbaum, W., & Kurth, W. (1967), *Genie, Irrsinn, und Ruhm: Genie-Mythus und Pathographie des Genies*, 6th ed. Munich: Reinhardt.

Lombroso, C. (1913), *The Man of Genius*, 3rd ed. London: Scott.

MacGregor, J. (1989), *The Discovery of the Art of the Insane*. Princeton, NJ: Princeton University Press.

Moebius, P. J. (1906), *Über Robert Schumanns Krankheit*. Halle: Marchold.

Monk, R. (1990), *Ludwig Wittgenstein: The Duty of Genius*. New York: Free Press.

Moreau, J.-J. (1859), *La Psychologie morbide dans ses rapports avec la philosophie de l'histoire*. Paris: Masson.

Nijinsky, V. (1913), *Notebook on "Life."* Typescript.

Nisbet, J. F. (1912), *The Insanity of Genius: and the General Inequality of Human Faculty Physiologically Considered*. London: Stanley Paul.

Ostwald, P. (1985), *Schumann: The Inner Voices of a Musical Genius*. Boston: Northeastern University Press.

—————— (1991a), *Vaslav Nijinsky: A Leap into Madness*. New York: Lyle Stuart (Carol Publishing Group).

—————— (1991b), Gustav Mahler from the viewpoint of psychoanalysis. In: *Das Gustav-Mahler-Fest Hamburg 1989; Bericht über den Internationalen Gustav-Mahler-Kongreβ*. Kassel: Bärenreiter.

—————— (1992), Psychotherapeutic facilitation of musical creativity. *Amer. J. Psychother.*, 46:383–404.

Pickering, C. (1974), *Creative Malady*. London: Oxford University Press.

Pollock, G. H. (1978), The mourning liberation process and creativity. *The Annual of Psychoanalysis*. New York: International Universities Press.

—————— (1990), Mourning through music: Gustav Mahler. In: *Psychoanalytic Explorations in Music: First Series*, ed. S. Feder, R. L. Karmel, & G. H. Pollock. Madison, CT: International Universities Press, pp. 321–339.

Reik, T. (1953), *The Haunting Melody: Psychoanalytic Experiences in Life and Music*. New York: Farrar, Straus & Young.

Rosen, C. (1991), Radical, conventional Mozart. *New York Review of Books*, Vol. 38, No. 21 (Dec. 19), pp. 51–58.

Rothenberg, A. (1990), *Creativity and Madness: New Findings and Old Stereotypes*. Baltimore & London: Johns Hopkins University Press.

Runyan, W. McK. (1982), *Life Histories and Psychobiography: Explorations in Theory and Method*. New York: Oxford University Press.

Schiller, F. (1982), *The Moebius Strip: Fin-de-Siecle Neuropsychiatry and Paul Moebius*. Berkeley, CA: University of California Press.

Singer, D. G., & Singer, J. L. (1990), *The House of Make-Believe: Children's Play and the Developing Imagination*. Cambridge, MA: Harvard University Press.

Solomon, M. (1977), *Beethoven*. New York: Schirmer.

—————— (1989), Franz Schubert and the Peacocks of Benvenuto Cellini. *19th Century Music*, 12:193–206.

—————— (1990), Mozart's Zoroastran riddles. In: *Psychoanalytic Explorations in Music: First Series*, ed. S. Feder, R. L. Karmel, & G. H. Pollock. Madison, CT: International Universities Press, pp. 401–421.

Sterba, E., & Sterba, R. (1954), *Beethoven and His Nephew: A Psychoanalytic Study of Their Relationship*, trans. W. R. Trask. New York: Pantheon.

Stevenson, R. L. (1886), *The Strange Case of Dr. Jekyll and Mr. Hyde*. London: Longmans, Green.

14

Eminent Mozart Performers' Panel

Clifford Cranna, Lise Deschamps Ostwald, Hans Hotter, Lotfi Mansouri, Paul Hersh, and Marc Gottlieb

Clifford Cranna: It is a great pleasure to be chairman for this panel discussion and to introduce the panelists who will do most of the talking, I hope. I'm giving you fairly detailed introductions to these people because I think that might be helpful when we get to questions from the floor in formulating your questions and directing them specifically to one of the panelists.

Two singers who were to have been with us today, Cheryl Parrish and Frederica von Stade, have had to cancel owing to illness and send their regrets. However, we were able to persuade a lady to join us, not wanting to be without one for this panel, and I'm grateful to her for stepping in on very short notice today. She can give us personal insight into what it's like to be a prodigious talent as a youngster. She was born in Montreal, Canada, the last of nine children, and started playing the piano in public at age 8. She won numerous awards and competitions, including a grant from the Canada Arts Council which allowed her to come to the U.S. to study with Egon Petri. In recent years she has created a program here in San Francisco called "Opera Go-Round" which is for young students. She recently produced a two-hour version of her own new translation of *The Magic Flute* which was performed with 100 students aged 10 to 12. It's a delight to have her with us. She has a family connection to our proceedings this afternoon, too: She is Lise Deschamps Ostwald. Thank you for being here.

191

Next, the gentleman on my left. It is a pleasure to introduce one of the great singers of this century: a bass-baritone who made his San Francisco Opera debut nearly forty years ago, in 1954, as the Flying Dutchman and in that same season sang a Mozart role, the Count in *The Marriage of Figaro*, and also Don Pizarro in *Fidelio*. He returned for many other seasons in subsequent years. A native of Germany, whose long career has included over 125 roles sung in all the major opera houses around the globe, he has been especially acclaimed for his performances of Wagner and is widely regarded as the foremost Wotan of his generation. He is still heard in occasional performances of such works as Schoenberg's *Gurrelieder* and many in this room, I am sure, heard his acclaimed portrayal of Schigolch in Lotfi Mansouri's production of Berg's *Lulu* in 1989. He has also enjoyed a career as a stage director and he still conducts a busy schedule of master classes around the world. We owe his presence in San Francisco now to that, as he is working with the Adler Fellows at the San Francisco Opera Center. And what a wonderful opportunity it must be for those young artists to work with the renowned Hans Hotter.

Next the gentleman on my far left: It's a pleasure to introduce my boss at San Francisco Opera, the general director there, a post he assumed in 1988. But he was no stranger to the Company then: He had been well known for many years in San Francisco, having served as stage director for literally dozens of opera productions at the War Memorial. He is a native of Iran, well-known now worldwide as a stage director. He staged productions at both the Zurich Opera and Geneva Opera in the 1960s. In 1976 he became general director of the Canadian Opera in Toronto, a post he maintained until coming to San Francisco. Among his many distinctions and innovations there was his use for the first time in North America of projected opera translations, which they call surtitles in Canada, and we persist in calling supertitles here in San Francisco.

He has worked with virtually all of the famous opera artists and has had a very special relationship over the years with Dame Joan Sutherland, directing her in no fewer than seven productions in San Francisco. Among the productions he has done for us here are the internationally telecast *La Gioconda* with Pavarotti; the 1988 telecast of *L'Africaine* with Domingo; Alban Berg's *Lulu* and last year's *Wozzeck* and also a new production of *Die Fledermaus*. This fall he brings us a new *Tristan und Isolde*. I should point out especially that he is chairman and instigator of the citywide festival we are now engaged in, "Mozart and His Time." And as I introduce him I should also point out that his name is often mispronounced—the T comes before the F—Mr. Lotfi Mansouri.

On my far right is a gentleman you have already heard from today in that remarkably interesting discussion of Mozart as performer. I don't need to say too much more about him, except for those who have just joined us. He is a distinguished musician, a very talented pianist, as most of you heard earlier, and an equally talented violist, on the faculty of the San Francisco Conservatory of Music, Mr. Paul Hersh.

And finally a gentleman who also brings us personal insight into what it's like to be extraordinarily talented as a youngster, in his case prodigy experience as a violinist. Currently resident conductor and principal concertmaster at the Tulsa Philharmonic, he has also served as resident conductor at the Kansas City Philharmonic. A native of Leipzig, he graduated from Juilliard and has performed widely throughout the United States as soloist and recitalist. He is also known as a lecturer and teacher and has conducted a number of artist residencies at various colleges and universities. The leader and founder of the renowned Claremont String Quartet, Mr. Marc Gottlieb.

Let me tell you a little about what I thought we might try to accomplish this afternoon. I'd like to steer the discussion in two primary directions, if I may. First, the idea of performing Mozart in general and of performing Mozart as a youngster, and secondly, what it's like to be a musical talent, an especially gifted musical talent, as a youngster. I'd like to start with the latter topic first, hoping we can have a little give and take around the table, and later open the discussion to questions from the floor.

Let's talk about what it's like to be talented, whether greatly so or moderately so, as a youngster. I'm going to throw that question first of all to you, Lise. Can you tell us a little about your experience?

Lise Deschamps Ostwald: My very early experience of Mozart is connected with a funny story. When I was 8 years old, I was auditioning and I was asked what I wanted to become, what I wanted to be when I grew up. And my answer to that was rather surprising for a child of 8 who was very small, very thin, very pale—you have to try to visualize that—my answer was "I want to be a Doctor in Music." The judges looked at me with smiles on their faces and said "Well, what will you play for us today?" I said I would like to play a Mozart sonata, the *Sonata in F Major* which has a lovely first movement but an even more beautiful second movement, very slow, expressive, with lots of ornaments, very lyrical, really my favorite movement. It also has a third movement, brilliant and fast and kind of fun to play. I enjoyed playing that.

After I played, one of the judges said, "You know, if you continue to play slow movements like that, I think you might get what you want, your Doctor." So now, looking back, I think he was right and wrong. I never did get a doctor's degree but I did get a doctor. I married one.

Clifford Cranna: When you realized you were very talented as a performer, how did that make you feel in relation to other children? Did you feel special? Did you feel isolated?

Lise Ostwald: I didn't think I had a special talent because I didn't know about such things. I was the ninth child and the only one who had a serious interest in music, but I also was very delicate and was not allowed by the doctors to jump or run or skip rope or play. So I really don't know what it's like as a child to play, except play piano, and this is why I enjoyed the last movement in that Mozart: I had an occasion to let my fingers run; that was okay, but *I* could not run. I never really went to school in a normal sense after I was 10 years old.

Cranna: Just like Mozart.

Lise Ostwald: Well, he never went to school at all. I enjoyed playing the works but I was not composing them as he was.

Cranna: Did you regret not being around other children, other students?

Lise Ostwald: No, but I think that's why now I enjoy working with students so much because it makes up for not having had that experience, and I relate very well with students.

Cranna: Marc, tell us about your experience as a child. Was it similar?

Marc Gottlieb: No. It really was not similar at all. When I was 4, my father gave me a little violin—which I still have—put it underneath my chin, and said "Play." And that's how it all started.

Cranna: Was this a Suzuki-type violin?

Gottlieb: No, this was in Germany and it was probably a German violin and I think it was an eighth-size with a little bow. And he said "Play" so I sort of took the bow and started to play. Now I have to tell you that my father was a violinist and my mother was a pianist and I had always heard music in the house, so for him to ask me or tell me to play was not that unusual. But basically for the rest of his life he didn't really tell me to do anything at all. He just really wanted me to study music and become a musician if I wanted to. I always, always, always wanted to be a baseball player.

I was a very small child—and there Lise and I do have a similarity—not even five feet tall when I was 15 and I weighed about 85 pounds. I was not undernourished but I certainly never ate very much. I played a lot of baseball and spent a lot of time out in the streets playing. Being a musician was really incidental in my life. I always knew I was going to be a musician, there was no question about that, but I also wanted to be a regular kid. I went to a lot of parties; I played a lot of ball; I practiced not all that much. Somehow or other I became a violinist; I don't really know how.

Cranna: Did you feel isolated?

Gottlieb: No, I never felt isolated from my contemporaries. I had a lot of friends, I socialized a lot, and I had a pretty good time.

Cranna: When did you make your actual debut as such?

Gottlieb: I actually made my debut as a violinist in Germany. I was tiny, tiny, and the concertmaster of the orchestra I played with was, I thought at the time, tall, tall, tall, though he was only 15 or 16 years old. I stood and played as concertmaster and he deferred to me and moved over and played as associate concertmaster. That's how I started to play.

My first experience with Mozart was not a particularly good one. I remember asking my mother, "Why does Mozart always end the same way?" and she said "I don't know what you mean." And I said: "It always ends (sings trill to tonic)." And she said to me, "Because he was a genius." And then she thought a little while and said, "You have to get a lot older to figure out what I mean."

Cranna: Thinking about a biography I read once of Yehudi Menuhin, who went through a sort of crisis of technique as a late teenager, having to relearn technical things that had come naturally earlier; I wonder, did you have an experience like that?

Gottlieb: I'm still having that experience. I always have crises in technique and I think I always will because it's sort of a natural phenomenon. You never really master what you want to do. That's one of the really great things about being a musician, I think. There's always the next day, the next hour, the next minute. You might discover something totally new and you might do something totally different from the way you've ever done it before.

Cranna: So practice doesn't diminish?

Gottlieb: No, it doesn't. Unfortunately I never practiced sufficiently but somehow I managed to get through. I really didn't discover what music was all about until I was about 30 years old. I did a lot of concertizing: I played 150 to 200 concerts a year starting when I was 21 or 22, but I didn't really know what music was about until I went to Marlboro and was initiated into the music phenomenon.

Cranna: So it's an ongoing process.

Gottlieb: Absolutely. And I've had many years to savor it and to love it.

Cranna: Paul, let's hear a little about your experiences as a youngster.

Paul Hersh: Mine are somewhat similar to yours, Marc. Both parents were musicians; my father used to get me out of bed at six in the morning to give me a violin lesson. We used to scream at each other, or so my mother says. And then I practiced piano in the afternoon. Did a little bit of playing but I really wasn't seriously into being a professional musician though I enjoyed playing a lot. When I went to college I didn't do any music at all except for playing in the symphony and playing quartets and stuff, and then I got this job with the Lenox Quartet quite by chance. They were recruiting my father to be the violist in the quartet but for one reason or another it didn't suit him so I said "I'd like to do that. I've always wanted to be in a string quartet." The Juilliard Quartet had kind of recommended me peripherally as being a talented dark horse or something. But I didn't even own a decent viola. I had this viola made by a local carpenter.

I remember that the cellist of their quartet wasn't in New York so I had to fly to Pittsburgh to audition. It was the first time I'd been on a plane since I was 4. I got to the audition place and the first thing they asked me was whether I played bridge or not. I said no. And they said "Well, if you're going to be in this string quartet you'll really have to learn to play bridge," and I agreed that would be okay. Then we had the audition. I remember we sat down and started to play and I think I lasted about ten minutes. I could see by the looks on my future colleagues' faces that what I was doing wasn't pleasing them in the least. They asked me "What is that viola?" I said, "Oh, I don't know; this is just something . . ."; "It sounds perfectly dreadful." Then one of them asked, "Isn't there a viola here?" Somebody said, "I think there is." There was one in the closet without any strings on it. They were quick to jury-rig it and hand it to me, and then they said, "Well, that sounds a little better."

"Look, you guys," I said, "I haven't played the viola very much but I'd really like to be in a string quartet and I'll practice all day long. . . ." I don't know why they did this. I thought for years afterward that they were probably wacko. I said to them, "If you want to audition me, I can't play all these notes, but take a short amount of music and show me what you want me to do and I'll try my best." I'll never forget: We worked for three hours up to the first double bar of the Haydn *Sunrise Quartet*. We got on that first note and I wasn't acceptable, I was just holding along on that first note, so we worked on that till it sounded pretty good and then we went on to the next note, and so it went. And I got the job!

I was in the middle of my junior year at Yale University doing an honors program in Western Intellectual History, so I came back to New Haven carrying 30 scores, from Carter and Schoenberg all the way back. I had to learn all of it. So I took a leave of absence for two years because their violist (the Lenox Quartet's) was leaving and going to the Claremont Quartet—so that's what I've been doing ever since. I took that job and I never went back to school. Later I got a college teaching job and went back to playing the piano.

Cranna: Was there any point when you were aware of being especially talented?

Hersh: Yes, I was talented as a kid but I didn't react well to performance pressure. Finally I decided I wouldn't be a musician because I got too nervous. I decided that when I was 13 or 14. I tried to play in public and it was a total disaster.

Cranna: I take it that subsided somewhat?

Hersh: Well, I have a strong feeling that it's not worth it if it's not fun. If it's not really joyous—there are so many other things one can do.

Cranna: Where did you make this transition?

Hersh: I decided I really wanted to play and took the means at my disposal to try to figure out why I got nervous. It might be interesting for this group—I went into psychoanalysis four times a week. I don't know that anyone would do that today.

Cranna: I hope you have good insurance.

Hersh: Well, it was cheaper then. I was a student.

Cranna: Mr. Hotter, can you tell us a bit about your early experiences? As a bass-baritone, I'm sure it was a while before you were aware of being able to sing or did you know that at an early age?

Hotter: Actually my mother told me that I had started to sing before I could speak, but that's just a silly remark. No, in fact I had not intended to become a singer. I had intended to become a musician, any field of music. I had worked in church music and had done an occasional solo before I met my later teacher. If I was to become a musician I had to learn something about singing, so it was only in order to learn more that I studied singing. I was already three years into a contract with an opera house before I really decided to stay with this profession.

Cranna: What age were you when you made your debut?

Hotter: I made my debut as an opera singer in 1930. I was 21.

Cranna: And you had no doubts after that?

Hotter: Certainly. As I said, it took me about four or five years until I made the final decision to stay or try to stay in this profession.

Cranna: Were there any regrets?

Hotter: No, actually not. But that comes with success. But I decided to do what my teacher always used to tell me: try to be a musician in the first place and a singer in the second place. I think if you are able to do this you will never lose interest.

Cranna: So in terms of your childhood experience there were no difficulties that made you wish you were not a musician?

Hotter: No, there were not. My father died when I was 7 years of age, and as a boy in school I was already singing soprano, but I took it for granted and didn't think there was anything . . . ingenious.

Cranna: What was a music education like in the schools at that time?

Hotter: Well, I didn't have music in the schools where I spent the early years of my education. Later on, after having finished high school, I was a member of the Musik Hochschule but not as a singer, as a pianist and organist.

Cranna: That's probably a little known fact. Lotfi, tell us, you began as a singer too, right?

Lotfi Mansouri: Very late in life. I was born in Iran and in Iran at that time music was not very much respected. In most of the families the ladies played a variety of musical instruments but men were not supposed to be musicians. I remember when I was young, about 14 or 15, I went to my father and said to him "I would love to play piano." And he said "Do you really like it?" I said, "I just love it." "Great," he said, "I'll pay somebody to play for you." That was the way it was. As a matter of fact, in the old Iranian language there was one word that all the musicians were called and it was not very complimentary. So my introduction to music at that time was in the films of Deanna Durbin. The first "Un bel di" I ever heard was Miss Durbin singing it in the film where she got her first kiss. But unfortunately she sang it in English. So that was my introduction to music until I came to the States, when I went to UCLA (University of California, Los Angeles).

Cranna: So the music that was performed in the homes mainly by the women was Iranian?

Mansouri: It was Iranian, not Western. My mother for instance played four different instruments. She played an Iranian instrument called Tar, like Sitar which is the three strings, and she studied violin for a long time. I learned to hate violin because it was so painful while she was practicing. For a long time I couldn't listen to violin until later when I started hearing people like Jascha Heifetz and then I realized, Hey, this is not bad. But most of the Iranians played Iranian instruments.

Cranna: So the decision to get into the musical world for you was relatively later.

Mansouri: I was a premed student. My father sent me to the United States to study medicine. The joke always goes that I saved a lot of lives by not becoming a doctor. When I was at UCLA as a premed, I was introduced to Western music and especially opera and that was like opening a whole new world for me. That all happened when I was about 19, 20, for the first time.

Cranna: So the idea of Western music, as contrasted with what was more customary in your homeland, was not a difficult transition for you.

Mansouri: No. Even as young man—perhaps it was the way my mother played those instruments—I never really liked the Iranian music very much. I always felt that anybody who was singing it must be suffering or in pain. The Iranian faster rhythms are wonderful: We have a percussion instrument called Dombek which is fabulous, a little bit like the South American percussion instruments. So I used to love the faster rhythms but the slower ones—I really thought they were souls in pain.

Cranna: So your entry into the opera world really came as a singer, is that right?

Mansouri: Actually my English then was even worse than it is now. I was studying all these heavy courses, physics, chemistry, and I was having a helluva time with a lot of homework. So my adviser said, "You should take a course that doesn't have any homework." So I said, "Well, what is there besides social dancing and boxing?" "You could take a chorus course, sing in a chorus." "Well, I don't know. I've never sung in my life." "All right, then, go a step back, start taking a voice class." So I took a voice class and my God! they found I had a voice. I was a tenor and I had a natural high C, no problem. The first aria they gave me to sing was "Che gelida manina." After I studied with voice teachers, I lost the high C. Actually from being a tenor I ended up. . . . I don't know where. We were talking about *Cosi fan tutte*: I have sung everything in *Cosi* except Despina. I started with Ferrando, then went to Guglielmo, and ended up as Don Alfonso, all with wonderful voice teachers.

Cranna: How did you become a stage director?

Mansouri: I'm a great believer in Kismet. In Iran Kismet means destiny. I was very much in demand: Tenors are always in great demand even if they're not good. I studied with Madame Lotte Lehmann; I even got a scholarship from her. She had twenty sopranos and I was the only tenor, so I got a chance to sing everything—Lohengrin,

Siegfried—everything she did. I was singing of all things, Sieg-
mund—I think you would have laughed a lot: I hate to go into this
story because it's very painful. The sword got stuck in the tree. There's
this wonderful line where he says "heraus aus der Scheide zu mir"
("Out of your sheath come to me") and I kept pulling but in rehearsals
the sword kept moving very loosely in the tree and didn't look as
though Papa had stuck it there. I told them, "Look, this has got to
stay a little stronger in there." So they put a hook on it, without telling
me. When I came to that line, I pulled and pulled on the damn thing
but it just wouldn't come out, so finally the whole tree came down.

Madame Lehmann said two wonderful things. One was to the
sopranos and mezzos she didn't like. Whenever they would get up
and sing something and she was really not very happy because she
knew they were not very good, she would say in a very kind way, "My
dear, why don't you go home and make babies." So when this happened to me, Madame Lehmann said, "Lotfi, have you considered
other options in opera besides singing?"

Then, as luck would have it, in one of the performances on stage,
I fell down and broke my left arm. It was a children's opera called
Tony Beaver: I don't think anybody has ever heard of it. I was one of
three farmers. In the opera there was a storm and a big flood and
the only way they could stop the flood was by putting kegs of molasses
and honey and following that with sacks of peanuts. Then all of a
sudden, of course, it all gets mixed up and you get peanut brittle. As
a farmer I had to jump up and go downstage to get some peanut
brittle. On the way I fell down and broke my left arm. After that,
they suggested that I try directing: "Lotfi, why don't you direct the
Prologue to *Ariadne auf Naxos*?" So that was it, that's how I started.

Cranna: Before we get to questions from the floor, I'd like to talk
more directly about performing Mozart. Lotfi, can you tell us a little
more about staging Mozart in your experience?

Mansouri: Of all operas in my life, the first professional job I had
was directing *Cosi fan tutte*. It was the first time I had really got paid
for directing something and I thought, Boy, this is easy; I know the
roles and all that. Now if you ask me to do *Cosi*, I am scared to death.
Because it is probably one of the most difficult, one of the richest,
most incredibly profound pieces of art that I've ever come in contact
with. Directing Mozart is very difficult because, especially in pieces
like *Magic Flute*, *Don Giovanni*, and *Cosi*, the problem is to find the

right balance. Let's take for example *Cosi*, as we're talking about it. If you go one inch toward too much comedy, you lose the truth, you lose the reality. If you go just a bit too much on the other side, you become solemn and ponderous and heavy. It is very difficult to find the correct balance in Mozart, where you deal with profound human relationships and issues but must not become pedantic or heavy. Same thing with *Don Giovanni*. He calls it a "dramma giocoso." You go one inch too far toward giocoso, you've lost it. You go a little too far toward drama, you've lost it. So to find that honest and true balance between those two sides is what scares me. When I'm faced with a Mozart opera, I'm always frightened about whether I'm going to find the right combination.

Cranna: Mr. Hotter, can you tell us about your experience in Mozart roles? Do they have special problems that you've experienced?

Hotter: No, I wouldn't say there are any special problems, except the problems you have always as a singer: to know, to use your work balance, to know how much do you have to act and how much do you sing. Or do you find a sort of a golden way in the middle where you can combine both? This seems to be mostly the problem with singers, as singers by nature are often not born artists: They are not musical sometimes, they are not actors; so they really have to try hard to find the way. To a certain extent you can learn these three things but if you are not gifted by nature, you have a hard time.

Cranna: Are there any differences you've noted between Mozart singing nowadays and when you were beginning your career? In the way Mozart is done or the kinds of singers who are doing Mozart?

Hotter: I wouldn't say there is any difference now, so far as Mozart is concerned. There may be a certain difference in how to sing today: Basically, I would say most of the young gifted singers try too early to be in the big operas with the leading roles. It takes a certain time to get used to these problems, to know how to act, to sing, to adjust yourself to your partners, to learn to watch the conductor without being too obviously caught looking down at him. Anyway, it takes a certain time, I would say at least five to eight years, before a singer would be ready to go into a leading part. And even if you are very gifted, a genius as a singer, today you are mostly too early.

It's very hard. Actually young singers need very much the advice of a qualified musician, a director, producer, conductor. . . .

Cranna: And a master teacher.

Hotter: I'm not one of those people who say everything was better fifty or eighty years ago, but I think definitely that the young singers of today have a harder time because there is a certain lack of qualified people in the musical field. Is that true?

Mansouri: Qualified technically you mean?

Hotter: No, I mean altogether. As I said, leading personalities such as directors, producers, conductors, with enough knowledge about what they should tell a young singer.

Mansouri: I completely agree. Because they don't go through their years of buildup, and experience, and getting enough knowledge.

Hotter: And this is what young singers need badly: to have somebody to advise them. Of course in the times where there was still ensemble opera, you had a contract with an opera house and had to stay there. As a young singer, you were not allowed to go away and give a guest performance. You had to stay in your own house. And there we had the elderly colleagues we could talk to; they could advise us. It was like the warmth of a nest where a bird grows up in this atmosphere. This the young singers are not offered, except to a limited extent, and for this I really wouldn't like to be a young singer today.

Cranna: Lise, what are your thoughts about performing Mozart? Special problems? Special things about it that have been part of your career?

Lise Ostwald: I think playing Mozart as a child was much easier than it is now. The older I get the more difficult it is I think to play Mozart well.

Cranna: There's an old saying about Mozart: especially for the piano, it's too difficult for adults and too easy for children.

Lise Ostwald: Yes, it's not only the fact that it's very transparent, one has to play very clearly, apparently it is quite simple and easy to memorize. But the complexities: The more you work on them, the more profound things you discover about Mozart. I could quote Liszt, who was talking about Chopin's Mazurkas, but it's also just as true of Mozart. Liszt said that those were wonderful miniature pieces but they were very deceptive, as is Mozart: "the canyon beneath the flowers."

Cranna: Marc, how about you? In the concerti—I presume you've done most if not all of them—do you find that they were written for an especially talented violinist? Do you get Mozart the violinist out of them?

Gottlieb: I always avoided playing Mozart whenever possible, because I really felt that I didn't know what I was doing, didn't know why I was doing it, and I always thought there was somebody else who could do it better than I.

Cranna: Was this out of a lack of affinity for the music itself?

Gottlieb: No, it was because I didn't trust myself. But there was an amazing breakthrough and it only happened about three years ago. I was asked to do a Mozart concerto as the soloist for a ballet company. I picked up the violin and somehow it was as though I'd played it all my life, I'd understood it all my life, loved it all my life, and will continue to love it. It was an amazing feeling to me to go out on the stage and play Mozart and be absolutely sure in my opinion, only my opinion, that it was absolutely right. I'm sort of happy with that. I hope the audiences were happy, too. I know the dancers were not. You know, they're counting one, two, three, four, in regular beats and you're doing it very differently. So you have to reconcile that. But I really didn't have too much trouble with that and I thought for the first time in my life that I had done a Mozart performance that I was pretty sure of.

Cranna: When we hear our violin auditions for the San Francisco Opera orchestra, we always require a Mozart concerto because it tells us a great deal about technique, in an instant.

Gottlieb: Correct. In my orchestral-experience life, I've sat in on—I don't know, I'll just throw out an obvious figure—a thousand violin and viola auditions. Everybody plays Mozart and they're all behind screens so I feel pretty safe in saying this: 99.99 percent of the Mozart concertos I hear are not very good.

Cranna: Why is that, do you think? What's lacking?

Gottlieb: I don't think those people have really come to grips with what they really have to do. Eventually, one hopes, something will happen to them as it happened to me, so that they become sure. Then comes another struggle, of course. Once you are sure of what you want to do, how sure are you *really* of what you want to do? But that's life. Tomorrow I might do it totally differently because I've been brought up to think that every performance should be different.

Cranna: That's the nature of art, isn't it?

Gottlieb: Yes, and every note should be different, and every time you touch something it should be different, so I'm not at all sure that tomorrow will be like I did it last year. But I was happy with what I did last year.

Cranna: Paul, tell us a bit about your performances of Mozart, both on piano and in chamber ensemble.

Hersh: I was going to say I think that one of the things that makes Mozart's music particularly difficult is that the margin for error is so very very slight. I liked Lotfi's talk about balance, because that balance for me is like being on a knife edge. The fewer the instruments the harder it gets. For instance, playing the piano concerti, which are very inspired pieces with a kind of dialogue between the orchestra and the piano, is a sheer delight. Playing the quartets and string quintets, which I do a lot, is similarly a delight. Playing the violin and piano sonatas—and this has been an interesting experience for me—in one's own small chamber with another fine musical colleague, is a great delight. But when you get on a stage especially in a large hall, those pieces become very very frustrating. Because the minute you try to project them, to send them across the footlights, I find that what happens is often inimical to what the music really requires. And lastly, playing the piano sonatas is something that I almost never do. I'm terrified of those pieces. Let me define my terms: You're driving in a car and you're a baseball nut like I am and the baseball game is on and you really want to turn to it except that when you flick on the radio, the classical music station has been left on from a previous trip, and something is being played, say a work of Mozart, and you *don't* switch to the ballgame. That's rare, for me. To play a Mozart piano sonata really well—I'm just being real bedrock honest—that's really rare. That is what I mean by good and that's a very high standard.

Someone asked me earlier about what recordings I'd recommend. I never used to read *High Fidelity* magazine, but one lunchtime I got my sandwich at the Conservatory and I grabbed it for something to read while I was eating. I read that a hundred critics had been asked for their favorite Mozart recording. This comprised all forms, opera, symphony, concerti, whatever, so those critics were not necessarily talking about the piano works. But guess what? In all those critical opinions there were only three pianists mentioned. If you had told me that ahead of time, I bet I could have guessed the artists and the performances. This is to me absolutely amazing. It certainly wouldn't happen with Beethoven or Schubert or Schumann because a lot of people play those pieces.

I'm sure you too can say what those choices were: Lipatti's recording of the A Minor Sonata (K. 310)—(we might totally disagree with this especially from any viewpoint of reasonable scholarship and performance practice, but it is merely magnificent); Fleischer's recording of the 503 (K. 503, N. 25 in C) with Szell and the Cleveland Orchestra, and the last one has to be that great performance of Schnabel with the New York Symphony or some such orchestra. The critic even points out that the orchestra is terrible. Schnabel drops all kinds of notes but the playing is incomparable. That is what I mean by good. And that is a terrifying standard to reach. You hear Mozart played a lot of the time and it just flows; it's so perfect and it's so even and it's so smooth and there's absolutely nothing to criticize—and you switch to the ballgame as fast as you can.

So what I'm saying is that with Romantic music like Beethoven and especially Schumann or Liszt, the standard is quite a different one from music which exists on a delicate balance, where to be fully engaged every spectrum of rhythm and of harmonic balance and proportion of the voices has to be achieved. Such a great performance, in Proust's description, is like a clear pane of glass: you don't notice it, you look at the landscape beyond. It brings opacities to that glass if the performance is not of that level.

Cranna: Intriguing remarks. A few things they stirred in my thoughts: One is a remark that a college professor of mine made and I've always remembered, quoting someone I suppose: that good Mozart is about as good as life gets. The other is a remark that Edo de Waart made in rehearsal, actually not of Mozart, but certainly applicable. It was that solo violin passage, Brunnhilde's awakening in *Siegfried*, which is so high and difficult, and he looked at the string players and said, "I know you're sitting in your nighties here." It's that feeling sometimes with Mozart: You're so exposed and there's no room for the slightest imperfection.

Hersh: I've never listened to a single Mozart tape or recording I've made and liked it. It's professionally acceptable, but I fear that one would go right to the ballgame.

Cranna: I want to throw out one general question that anybody can grab at. It has to do with the state of education, of music education in our country today. If a Mozart appeared amongst us at the age of 4 or 6 or 8, what could we expect to happen? Would we ever recognize him? Is he perhaps amongst us? Would he even go into music? Any takers on that? Any thoughts?

Mansouri: He might have to be packaged.

Cranna: He'd need an agent.

Mansouri: With a multimedia contract and lots of publicity and agents and all the rest because nowadays the music business has become so unbelievably commercial. You can imagine what would happen to Mozart if he came today. One of the agents would get hold of him and one of the record companies and they would be packaging him, and have the publicity machines going and everything else, so that's what is a little bit frightening about our time now.

Cranna: Do you think he would be steered into the area of virtuoso performing rather than composing?

Mansouri: Whatever made the most money.

Cranna: Then obviously into performing. Any other thoughts on that?

Gottlieb: I would think he'd wind up in Hollywood. And write a lot of fast music. One day this, and tomorrow that. I think it would be almost impossible for a Mozart as we know him to grow up and exist and write 622 or 750 works and have them eventually performed. We can see by what's happening to the composers of today. Nobody writes that amount and they all struggle to get things performed. I don't think any of us has the time to wait 250 years to find out what's going to happen.

Hersh: Would it be unreasonable to suggest that what Mozart was subjected to and seemed not to find great displeasure in, is extraordinary even to our imagination today? Traveling around year after year under those conditions, being made to perform every day, being a kind of a lapdog to the aristocracy: These are most fearsome and unnatural situations for a small child, it seems to me. I think that the packaging might be a relief; at least one would not have to sit in the coach.

And Mozart was sick a good deal of the time: There were frequent epidemics and when people got sick, it was for a long time. There's that story from his early time in Vienna when there was a typhoid epidemic. Leopold came and literally lifted Wolfgang out of Vienna. He left the ladies there but he and Wolfgang took off. They are kind of horrific stories.

The more I read about Mozart as performer, the more I get into the source material, the more I realize that he was one of the most extraordinary performers of all time. Somebody said, was it Haydn, that we won't see his like for another hundred years. I don't think we have. He seems to have been a kind of autistic child of music: He could do extraordinary things that just defy the imagination.

Cranna: So you think we may not see another one?

Gottlieb: I think life today doesn't allow another Mozart to come up.

Hersh: I think not. That's individual genius, don't you think?

Gottlieb: Of course it's individual genius and there might be many individual geniuses among us but to reap the benefits of that type of genius is very difficult to do in today's world. I'm sorry to be negative about that.

Cranna: I'm going to open it up to questions now.

Questioner: Have you ever had what could be called a religious experience playing Mozart or hearing Mozart performed?

Hersh: Could I just ask the questioner to define what he means by religious experience?

Questioner: You define it for yourself. It's fascinating, as described earlier, that Mozart always seemed to be going from the mundane, the experience of life in the present with feet on the ground, to things that were truly transcendental. So I guess it's the transcendental experience I'm asking about.

Mansouri: I could answer, for myself only. If you mean by religious experience something beyond the daily norm of life, something that's very profound and on a level that you can't really even describe, for me it happened when I was doing the Trio in the first act of *Cosi fan* *tutte*: Fiordiligi, Dorabella, and Don Alfonso. Once when I was directing it, I felt such a real intertwining of lives, experiences, emotions, everything involved in it, that it was as if time stopped. All of a sudden you felt very grateful to have the opportunity to confront such a piece; you felt that all the years that you had worked were worth it. Now every time I hear this trio—and it happened again the other day in a rehearsal—I feel exactly the same way: a kind of total uplifting and total suspension, even from reality.

Lise Ostwald: I also had a very moving experience. I wouldn't call it really a religious experience. My husband can confirm this. We were in Leipzig—that was already a very interesting situation because we were there for a festival on Schumann and Peter happened to have grown up in an area where his grandparents' house was still standing, so the whole city had a lot of meaning for us—we were invited to attend a concert at the Gewandhaus which was conducted by Kurt Masur and the soloist was Emil Gilels. I have strong admiration for Emil Gilels. I wouldn't say that he's my favorite pianist: I've heard him do things that I did not like. But this particular performance was the last Mozart piano concerto, the B flat (K. 595). The first movement was beautifully played; the second movement was an experience such as you have once in a lifetime. I don't know if the word *religious* is appropriate for that. I was so moved by the sound that came out, the incredible suffering that appeared on this man's face as he was performing this movement, that I was actually crying and I turned to my husband. There were tears on his face also so I thought, I'm not the only one who is responding this way.

Hersh: Sometimes Mozart can be very refreshing. I remember an experience while my wife and I were traveling through Europe. We were just looking at visual arts, no sounds. We got back to London and she turned on the radio. I hadn't heard any music for two weeks and a piece came on that I used to play with my parents and have played many many times, almost to the point of it's being too much. It's the Kegelstadt Trio, clarinet, viola, and piano (K. 498). That came on the radio and it would be very difficult to describe how beautiful that sounded. It was just deep and beautiful and transcendent, in the sense that I didn't listen with the usual professional things that crop up in my mind: Is that being well played? Who is that? those kinds of questions. It was just straight to the heart of those very simple and perfect lines. Also, I would say the piece sounded reborn: It was as though I had never heard it before. So the new context established a kind of truth and greatness in that music which I hadn't suspected.

One of the troubles about listening to Mozart—and I think it's even more of a problem with the instrumental music than it is with the vocal music, especially the piano music—is that the sense of nuance needs to be reasserted. You have to feel the difference in one note as opposed to the next, or an articulation or a particular rhythmic accent, so one of the good things about talking about Mozart, about getting together and sharing it, is that it suggests a level of excitement and perhaps enthusiasm for the small and for the simple, not for the grand and the sock-you-between-the-eyes kind of thing. I think that's a really good thing. If there's anything we lose in the mass media, I think it's that sense and awareness of detail. Who was it who said "God is in the details?" That's one of the good things about getting attuned.

Questioner: I have a question about the nuance in Mozart that Mr. Hersh was talking about. What is Mozart looking for when he indicates, as in the adagio in B minor, "sforzando," which he uses a lot in that piece. Is he looking for something suddenly loud, or an accent, or what? I would like to hear you talk about that, or is this more for a master class on nuance?

Hersh: There are four kinds of strong accents in Mozart. Going all the way at times from the dot, which is the most subtle separation of a note from its neighbors, practically closest to the legato; then the wedge, which indicates a more clarified separation, the sforzando piano, which indicates a gentler and more immediate backing off from the strong, and then the sforzando, which to me, even though it would be governed by its context, would be the strongest expression of emphasis. A sforzando in Mozart is not quite the same as a sforzando in Beethoven, in my view. In Beethoven the sforzando is really more of a moment of surprise and in Mozart it may be a more gentle and searching emphasis, more like a scooped shape rather than a quick and hard chop.

Questioner: Where did he get that? Is it not a classical mark?

Cranna: It's a pianistic device which comes along with the classical period.

Questioner: There have been allusions made to the Catholicism of Mozart's family. And yet we know that *The Magic Flute* has a basis in

Freemasonry and he composed a lot of other music for Freemasonry. I'm curious as to what his connection with Freemasonry was and how it affected his music.

Hersh: Some of my graduate students did a big study project on the number three and the relationship to the Masonic symbols and the use of three notes, but again I think this is more a question for scholars than for performers.

Cranna: There's a wealth of speculation to be made about that, not only with relation to *The Magic Flute* but a great deal of the other music as well.

Questioner: A question to Mr. Mansouri. Now that we are playing Mozart on original instruments, are there efforts to perform Mozart operas in what is known of style of the period?

Mansouri: Unless you are creating productions for historical interest and you want to go back and try to re-create the style of the period, I don't see much value in it personally. I always get a little impatient when people talk about something "in the original style of Mozart." Who the hell is around now who was there to bring it back and tell us what the Mozart style was? Even if you talk about the original instrumentation, you don't have the original acoustics, you don't have the original halls, so it is for me a rather fruitless effort. There are a lot of people who delight in it and would like to re-create it. I don't think you can totally re-create it: I wasn't there, I don't know what it sounded like at that time. I don't know anyone who was. So how would you judge it? If you are doing scholarly research, that's one thing. In performance the most important thing is the communication to the audience you're playing to. In *Cosi fan tutte* or *The Marriage of Figaro*, I don't know what you would add with original instruments.

There's very little documentation of the staging style. If you saw the *Amadeus* film, for example, the excerpts they did of *The Marriage of Figaro* and some of the others, they were not authentic at all. They were danced in some cases and there was a kind of interpretation of that particular style. When I was studying at the Music Academy of the West, we had a director, Dr. Herbert Graf, who was a very well-known director from the Metropolitan Opera, and he did re-create *The Magic Flute* in the original designs of its world premiere. As a matter of fact, I had the wonderful opportunity of playing and singing Monostatos in it. But it was just as a background. It had things like that wonderful drop with the stars for the Queen of the Night—I think you can find that now. That has stayed. I've never been really involved in any of the performances that have tried to strive for that authenticity.

Cranna: There would be enormous problems, obviously, just in trying to re-create the atmosphere. But one has to remember that the audience in Mozart's day didn't sit in the dark as we do. The lights were on and the whole idea of dimming the lights and creating those magical effects onstage was quite a bit different. We have vastly different expectations about what we're going to see.

Questioner: Mr. Mansouri, what do you think of the balance that has been maintained or not maintained by modern productions, particularly in the Peter Sellars ones we've seen.

Mansouri: I'm going to talk only about my personal reactions. I watched the *Don Giovanni* of Mr. Sellars and as I was watching it I had a very strange feeling that I was watching one channel for visual things and I was hearing something else. What I was hearing was not correlating with what I was seeing. When, for example, I was hearing sung in Italian "questo piatto saporito," "this deliciously tasty dish," and I saw the Big Mac and the Fries, I felt maybe I'm listening to the wrong channel. So I think it's amusing, it's fun, but I don't know what it adds, to tell you the honest truth, in *Don Giovanni* when you have twin brothers playing the Don and Leporello and you have Donna Anna shooting some coke before her aria. I'm not a fan of that kind of thing because I don't think it adds to the understanding. Mozart has been dealt with in so many ways and it has survived all those ways and it will probably survive this, too. But at the same time I think it's interesting to see it done differently. It's like doing Shakespeare. For me Mozart is like what Shakespeare is to theater. Because you can do Shakespeare's plays in any variety of periods, costumes, interpretations, and it's so rich, it has so much value, that you can always find so much in it. I feel the same way about Mozart operas. You can do *Don Giovanni* in hundreds of different ways and look at it through the different prisms of the interpreters, of the directors, and all that. Some could be valid or not valid, but everybody must find what's good for them. I personally didn't think that production of *Don Giovanni* added anything to my love or appreciation of the opera.

Questioner: I'd like to address a question to Professor Hotter. In psychology a good deal has been written about the difference in emotional expression through speech and through singing. You have experience in both spoken and sung roles on the stage, I wonder if you'd share with us some of your own feelings about whether that's a different experience for you. What is it like for a singer to take a speaking role, in terms of the kinds of emotional expression that are involved in projecting the role?

Hotter: Phonetically it's practically the same. A throat doctor once explained to me that the processes of speaking and singing are identical. The only difference is that the vocal chords when you speak vibrate only with the inner edges. When you sing the whole chord vibrates. This is physiologically the explanation that singing and speaking should come from the same origin. But there is one thing that is so much neglected in our time: that the young singers do not learn equally to speak in addition to the singing. So if you really know how to use your voice, you can equally speak and sing. And it's up to your own feeling and your own liking whether you prefer one or the other. There is no difference in fact as an artistic production.

Questioner: But there are some people who are able to sing—people who have aphasia, for example: They may be able to sing something but they can't get it into words.

Cranna: Is that because there's a different mental process involved? We're talking about people who can't speak for some reason although they can sing.

Mansouri: Also emotional. One artist I worked with stuttered very markedly when he spoke but when he sang it was absolutely clear; there was no difficulty and not the slightest stutter. I attributed that more to emotional causes, certain fixations, rather than to physical ones.

Questioner: Mr. Mansouri, I'm curious to know how your father reacted when he learned that you had given up medicine for music.

Mansouri: He disowned me. It was rather sad for me because we did not communicate for twenty years. When the Shah of Iran built an opera house in Teheran, he invited me to go back and do some organization, and then I had a wonderful reunion with my father.

Questioner: This is to all of you. When performing, have you ever had an experience where you seem to take on another personality or a personality beyond your usual workaday world?

Mansouri: I can say that in opera you can't do that because you've got to be so much aware of the musical values: rhythm, notes, pitch, dynamics, orchestra, and others. I have a feeling that if you did take on another personality you'd get completely out of connection with the conductor and would have to stop. I can't imagine that kind of departure happening in opera. It has happened in theater, I know, that some actors have been so emotionally involved in their roles that for short periods of time they have identified completely with the characters they were playing rather than themselves.

Hotter: May I add a story out of the experience of my wife? When we were newly married, my wife invited one of her school friends to hear an opera because she said, "Now that I'm married to an opera singer we should go." I was doing Pizarro in *Fidelio*. My wife told her friend, "My husband plays a lot of villains." And the girl said, "Doesn't that have an influence on his private life?" So that explains the other personality.

Cranna: What about all the times you have performed Wotan? Did you ever feel that you were changing, taking on a different persona as Wotan?

Hotter: I had an enormously great experience when I was a young singer, seeing and hearing Feodor Chaliapin on the stage. At that time—it was the early thirties—he was actually, I think, among the few very great actors on the operatic stage. I read his biography and in it he said, "I'm not supposed to turn into this or that character. I only have to try to project whatever I want to say about him. I'm not going to be the person myself."

During the first week or two of rehearsal, I may try to be the person himself but after a while I step out of him and watch myself. It's not I who has to have a mood, or a particular quality. It's the audience who should be moved, not me. But I have to project all the things which bring the audience to the understanding of that personality.

Hersh: I think that's very well put. It's not the character, it's the idea of the character that one is projecting. To project the idea requires a full consciousness of who one is and who that character is. Otherwise you don't achieve the absolute beginning idea of dramatic art which is that projection, I think.

Questioner: Is there a lot of difference between Stanislavski and Brechtian acting techniques?

Cranna: Do those apply, do you think, to operatic acting?

Mansouri: Do you mean Brecht in his anti-illusion, and Stanislavski in creating the illusion? Yes, with Stanislavski the idea was that you dealt so much with the personality and the character that you were playing that you created the illusion of being that person. With Brecht the idea was that he wanted to break the illusion. If you remember any real Brechtian staging, it was done with incredibly strong white light. He wanted very much to break the distance between the audience and the performer so you do not have that barrier and that kind of division.

Questioner: Is it still taught?

Mansouri: Yes, in theater classes, in acting classes. As you know, the Stanislavski method was the basis of so-called Method acting in New York and all that. But for better or worse you can't use that in opera because opera has its own exigencies. A perfect example of Method acting was Marlon Brando: If you asked him how are you, he had to kind of wait, delve into the past and all the characters and everything that had happened before he could answer, or grunt, "Fine." If you did that in opera, the music would be two or three pages ahead of you by the time you got the words out. So it's a different technique.

Questioner: Mr. Hotter, could you talk a bit more about this idea of stepping out of yourself? You mentioned when you were rehearsing. . . .

Hotter: I think a young artist, a young singer in this case, would always try to imagine that "I *am* the person" very individually. The more you grow, the more mature you become, the more you will try to separate your being from what you do. You sort of learn to watch yourself and think of the movements you should make. When I was a young singer, I found I was doing this, for instance (arm gesture) and I said, "How do I get rid of this? How do I get it down?" And a friend said, "All you do is to use your left hand and drop the other."

That was right: Everybody looked at the left hand. There is the technique and certain tricks you have to learn. At the beginning you are not aware of what you do and then after a while, with the help of good producers and directors, you will learn to be in control of your acting and at the same time to watch your voice. It is a double or actually a triple job you have to do: the language, the voice, the speaking, the conductor, the colleagues. If you try to take all of this apart, you are lost.

Cranna: I was trying to think of a way to conclude our deliberations about Mozart and I thought of the question some have raised, some critics especially, "Are we going too far with all this? This year, with all the Mozart mania?" And I ran across the perfect remark about that by David Cairns, the critic of the London *Sunday Times*, writing in the San Francisco Opera program magazine. He said, "Mozart is the most human as well as the most celestial of the great composers, whose depth we shall never fathom and whose variety we will not exhaust, even in 1991."

Name Index

Subject Index